The Recipe to Life

AF896473

Bridgette Flagg

Copyright © 2026 By Bridgette Flagg

All Rights Reserved.

Table of Contents

Dedication

First, I would like to thank you, God, for all you have done. Your grace and mercy you have shown me my entire life.

I dedicate this book to myself. Writing this took courage, strength, and a lot of grace. I've been working on this book for years, starting over, stopping, doubting myself, and sometimes not believing I was even capable of finishing it. There were moments I wanted to give up, moments I felt stuck, and moments I didn't believe in myself at all. So, this book is for the new version of me, the woman who kept going anyway. And it's also an apology to the old version of me. I did the best I could with what I had, and now I give myself grace.

Secondly, I dedicate this book to my mother, my grandmother, and my father. I miss you more than words can explain. I carry you with me in everything I do. Thank you for your love, your sacrifices, and the foundation you gave me. I hope you're watching over me. I hope I'm making you proud.

Lastly, I dedicate this book to my family, my sisters, and most importantly, my children. I hope this book helps you understand who I am and the road I've had to walk. Every sacrifice I made, every bad decision, every late night and tear was for you. Everything I do is for you.

Bryan and Brielle, you are my why. I love you beyond words.

Acknowledgment

I would like to express my deepest gratitude to everyone who helped bring The Recipe To Life *to life. To my visual team, Sharday McCollough, Rob Sese, and Charles Thomas, y'all made this book shine with every photo and design.*

To Racquel Peacher, thank you for never stopping, for always answering when I called in my time of need while trying to put these words on paper. Your patience and support meant more than you know.

To my family and friends, thank you for your love, encouragement, and constant support throughout this journey.

And to my readers, thank you for taking this journey with me. This book is for you, from my heart to your table.

About the Author

Bridgette Flagg is a Chicago-based restaurant owner, community leader, and first-time author. She is the owner of **Soulè Chicago** *in North Lawndale and* **Soulè to Soulè** *in Ukrainian Village, and the founder of the* **Soulè Cares Foundation**, *a nonprofit focused on feeding families, uplifting communities, and giving back with purpose.*

The Recipe to Life *is not a traditional cookbook. It is a collection of real stories, hard lessons, and healing moments told through food. Each recipe represents a chapter of Bridgette's life, the loss, the mistakes, the growth, the faith, and the resilience it took to become the woman she is today.*

Raised in Chicago, Bridgette learned early that food brings people together. What started in her mother's kitchen turned into a passion, a business, and now a book. Writing The Recipe to Life *was part of her healing journey, a promise she made to herself and to God to tell her story honestly and walk in her purpose.*

Through her restaurants, foundation, and now her writing, Bridgette's mission is simple: to feed people, inspire healing, and show that no matter where you come from, transformation is possible.

In The Recipe to Life, *Bridgette Flagg blends personal stories with cherished recipes, weaving together moments of struggle, faith, and triumph. This book is more than just a cookbook; it's a testament to resilience, healing, and the power of food to bring people together. Join Bridgette on this heartfelt journey of transformation and inspiration.*

Prelude

From the busy streets of Chicago to the heart of Soulè, my journey has been anything but ordinary. *The Recipe to Life* isn't just about cooking; it's about the real stories behind each dish, stories of resilience, love, and transformation.

Growing up, the kitchen was my safe haven. It's where I found my purpose, and where meals brought people together. Each chapter in this book reflects a chapter of my life, the ups and downs, the struggles and victories, the moments of doubt, and the power of faith.

In these pages, you'll get more than just recipes; you'll get a piece of my heart and the journey that shaped each dish. This prelude is an invitation to walk with me through the flavors of my past and the hope that guided me forward.

Welcome to the kitchen of my life. Let's create something extraordinary together.

Introduction – The Recipe to Life

Being from the Westside streets of Chicago, you see so much chaos daily, including killings, drug dealing, and drug abuse. Physical and mental abuse was also served on too many people's plates.

I knew early on that I didn't want that life to be my future. My mom, dad, and grandmother did everything in their power to make sure we were good, and for the most part, they kept us afloat. Back then, we didn't have social media to compare our lives to others'. We knew we were struggling, but it didn't hit as hard because we weren't constantly reminded of what we didn't have.

As time went on, I started losing the very people who grounded me: first, my father, then my grandmother, and eventually, my mother. I found myself in this world just trying to survive.

When you grow up in certain environments, it's easy to fall into habits you're not proud of. I tried my best to stay on the right path, but eventually, I became a product of my surroundings. I started doing things just to keep up with the people, with the lifestyle, with the pressure. I faced physical and mental abuse, depression, loneliness, just running from my reality, and making reckless decisions.

At the rate I was going, I was headed two places, and

neither one was heaven. Jail or Hell.

This book is *The Recipe to Life*.

Each story unwraps a part of my journey, and every recipe ties back to a moment in time that helped shape who I am. I pray that through these stories and flavors, you get a deeper taste of my truth.

I hope you enjoy.

The Dumbo – Gumbo Recipe

Growing up, my mom and dad always made sure we had everything we needed and a lot of what we wanted. We lived in a 17-room house, complete with a toy room, a dungeon, and even a wine cellar. My sister had a car when she couldn't even drive yet. We had it all: the parties, the lifestyle, the attention. My mom and dad had plenty of friends, and let's just say, they were "in the business."

Eventually, though, drugs took over my father's life. My mom, who had always been more of a housewife than a worker, wasn't prepared for the shift. Everything started to slow down. But if you've ever lived a certain kind of way, you know the show must go on, by any means necessary.

I went off to Jackson State University for a couple of years, but when I came back home, my life took a turn. I met a guy from out of state at one of Chicago's hottest Tuesday night parties, The Buzz. He was charming, flashy, and different. He introduced me to fine dining, weekend trips, and street life. My mother wasn't a fan. She knew something wasn't right about him, but I couldn't see it. I was head over heels.

I was in what I call the *"lies and butterflies"* stage of my life. Everything felt perfect on the surface, but I was ignoring all the red flags. That all changed the day I got a call from my brother.

"Go check on Daddy," he said. "He didn't show up to work."

That alone shook me. My father *never* missed work, not even after he was diagnosed with cancer of the larynx, not even through addiction, not even through the streets. He was a man who never let life stop him.

I rushed to his building on the West Side, owned by a man who also owned Shine King, the legendary shoe repair shop. I asked him to let me into my dad's apartment.

As I walked up to the third floor, a foul smell hit me hard. My nerves were already a mess. Thank God the odor wasn't coming from my father's unit, but somewhere else. Still, I knew something wasn't right.

His gate had no lock. The door was open. That wasn't like my father. He always kept things locked up, no matter what.

I called his name.

No answer.

I was too scared to go in. I asked the man to check for me. A moment later, he came out, shaking his head. *No.*

I ran in.

And there he was, my father, lying still in bed. Lifeless. His eyes were gray. His face was still wet from tears that had rolled down his cheek.

It was like the world stopped spinning.

Seeing how he died and *how he was living* broke something in me. From a 17-room house to a tiny studio apartment. From everything to… this.

From having it all to that dark, lonely studio apartment, it wasn't just sad; it was crawling with rodents, and it was nothing like the life he should've had. I still cry, because I feel like he died in that room, alone. He'd left drugs behind, but alcohol took hold. And deep down, I knew someone had robbed and killed him. His cancer wasn't that advanced. When I found him, his trach was missing. His door was unlocked. I told the police that this wasn't normal. But they did nothing. They just put him in a black bag. When they called it cancer, no autopsy, my heart shattered. I knew there was more. But all I had left was grief.

Laying my father to rest broke something deep inside me. I was his baby girl, and suddenly, I had to plan a funeral, something I never imagined doing. I picked his suit, wrote his obituary, and chose every flower, determined to honor him fully. As a veteran, he had the 21-gun salute, but none of it eased the ache. At his casket, I stood remembering how much he loved me, how he bragged that I was his first child to go to college, how I could do no wrong in his eyes. I couldn't stop touching his face; it was cold, and I can still feel it to this day. My first true love, my father, was gone.

I was angry. I was devastated. I was lost. And in that pain, I ran. I ran straight into the arms of the man I thought loved me. The one who offered me a way out, even if that "way out" was really a deeper trap.

We hit the streets together. I was traveling to Texas, New York, moving weight, and making money. But deep down, I knew it wasn't the life I wanted. I begged him to stop. I told him I wanted to go back to school, to live a normal life. He promised me, *"One last run."*

Only this time, he tried to send me alone with some girl I barely knew. I wasn't having it. "If we're doing this, we're doing it together," I told him. We were supposed to be like Bonnie and Clyde, after all, or so I thought.

He agreed.

We made the transaction in Texas. I waited for him in the hotel. Hours passed. No word. No calls. Finally, he picked up. "I'm at the airport," he said casually. "You'll have to ride back with the girl."

My heart dropped. *What?!*

I was furious. Hurt. Scared. But I had no choice. It was my rental car, my product, bought with the money my father left me. My investment in a better life.

The entire ride back, I prayed, *"Lord, please get me back to Chicago. Please don't let me go to jail."*

When we made it back, I noticed we were taking the exit to *his* house. Confused, I asked, "Where are we going?" The girl said, "Right here."

We pulled over. He was standing there, waiting.

She unlocked the doors. He took all of my product out of the car.

"I got a sale," he said.

I screamed, "Are you serious? That's mine!"

Long story short… he robbed me. I never got a return on my investment. He claimed he got robbed. And as crazy as it sounds, that was only the beginning of a toxic, painful, and draining relationship.

Still to this day, I thank God for His mercy and favor. I was living wild, blinded by pain and love, running from a reality I didn't know how to face. And yet, God kept me.

This gumbo, this messy, bold, chaotic, spicy dish, is a reflection of that time in my life. A little bit of everything, thrown into one pot: grief, survival, betrayal, heartbreak, and a whole lot of seasoning.

Gumbo

Ingredients

The Trinity & Veggies

- 3 cups celery, chopped
- 3 cups okra, sliced (fresh or frozen)
- 3 cups red & green bell peppers, mixed
- 3 cups white onion, chopped
- 1 tablespoon green onion (for garnish)
- 1 teaspoon parsley (for garnish)
- 3 bay leaves

Seasonings

- 2 tablespoons celery salt
- 2 tablespoons celery seeds
- 2 tablespoons gumbo filé
- 2 tablespoons cayenne pepper
- 1 tablespoon Cajun seasoning
- 2 tablespoons Creole seasoning
- 2 tablespoons Soulè Secret Seasoning

- 3 tablespoons chicken soup base

Liquids

- 1 cup Worcestershire sauce
- ½ cup hot sauce

Proteins

- 4 boneless chicken breasts
- 2 packs blackened chicken sausage, sliced
- 4 crab leg claws

For the Roux

- 2 sticks of butter
- 1 cup flour
- 2 teaspoons minced garlic
- 1 teaspoon Creole seasoning

Instructions

Whew **chileeeee**… I already know what y'all are thinking, because I was thinking the same thing while writing all this down. It sounds like a lot, but trust me, these are basic staples you want in your cabinet anyway.

1. Cook the Chicken

Start by boiling the chicken breasts in a **16-quart stock pot** (it doesn't *have* to be that big, but this recipe is based on that size).

Once fully cooked, remove the chicken, **reserve the broth**, shred the chicken, and place it back into the pot with the broth.

2. Build the Gumbo Base

Add the sliced okra (frozen is perfectly fine), sliced sausage, and crab leg claws to the pot.

Then add:

- Bay leaves
- Celery
- Okra
- Bell peppers
- White onion

3. **Season It Right**

Sprinkle in:

- Celery seeds
- Celery salt
- Cayenne pepper

- Cajun seasoning
- Creole seasoning
- Chicken soup base
- Soulè Secret Seasoning

Stir everything together, then let it simmer over medium heat.

4. Make the Roux

In a separate saucepan, melt **2 sticks of butter** over medium heat.

Add minced garlic and Creole seasoning.

Once it starts bubbling, whisk in the flour slowly.

Keep whisking until the roux is smooth and consistent; no lumps.

5. Bring It All Together

Pour the roux into the gumbo pot and stir well.

Let the gumbo **boil on medium heat for about 45 minutes**, stirring occasionally. Add water if needed.

6. Serve & Garnish

Once done, ladle into bowls and garnish with green onion and parsley.

And just like that… there you have it: **Gumbo.**

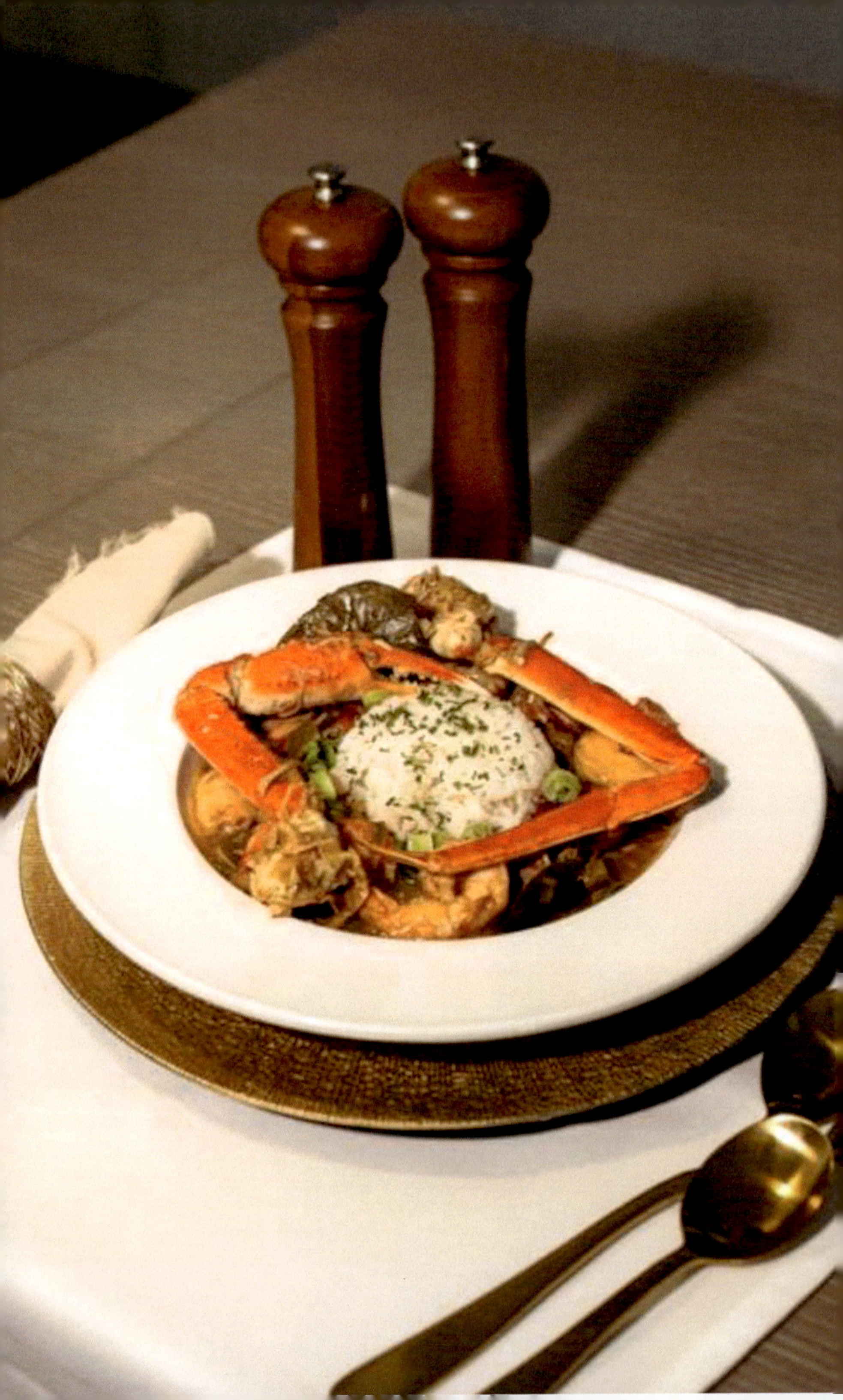

Feeling Smothered – Smothered Chicken

I really thought I would be over him after he robbed me and took my money. I told myself that was it, that I was done. But that wasn't the case.

He swindled his way right back in with trips, gifts, and dinners. Money was still coming in, just not the way it used to. He would piece it back little by little, a few hundred here and there, just enough to keep me quiet, just enough to keep me hoping.

What I didn't know was that this man was living a whole double life.

One day, I watched him put in his voicemail code. I don't even know why I paid attention, but after that moment, I had access. That's when everything unraveled. Voicemails from women I'd never heard of. People calling, looking for him. Threats on his life. That's when I realized, it wasn't just me. I wasn't special. I wasn't the only one he had fooled. I had been dating a stranger.

Still trying to hold it together, I bought a brand-new Dodge Charger. In my mind, life was going okay, or at least I was pretending it was.

One day, he asked to use my car, and like a fool, I let him. That same day, I had to take my grandmother back to the nursing home. She had suffered a bad stroke and was living there, but they allowed her to come home for the weekend. Seeing her back in her own bed, in her own house, felt like old times. She couldn't talk, but the joy on her face said everything. I was soaking in every moment, not knowing how important that day would become.

Hours went by. He was still gone. I started calling. Over and over. More than 30 times. No answer. When he finally picked up, he told me he wasn't bringing the car back. I panicked. A few friends and I started riding around the city, hoping to spot the car because the color stood out. When we finally found him, it turned into a real-life standoff. He was so angry that he broke the key off in the ignition.

I was devastated, but not just about the car.

I had to take my grandmother back to that nursing home, back to that place that felt like a hellhole to me. I didn't understand how I let a man put me in this position. I didn't understand the hold he had on me.

All I could think about was my father.

I had recently lost him. I was a daddy's girl; I was his world. His love was unmatched. And without realizing it, I was chasing that love. I wanted to feel protected, wanted, chosen. I wanted to feel loved again, and I kept looking for it in the wrong man.

He cried. He apologized. He told me he was dealing

with things. He told me he loved me. He promised to do better. And I believed him; I believed every word. He knew exactly how to play on my heart.

I told myself I would never let him use my car again.

And then I did.

"Baby, I need to bust a move real fast. I gotta go pick up some money."

Hours passed. No call. I called him.

"Hey, babe, where you at?"

"I had to run to New York real quick. I'll be back."

New York? I needed my car. I had to work. Before I could even react, he hung up. I didn't call the police. I couldn't bring myself to do it. This was my man. I loved him. I couldn't believe he would do me like that.

But he did.

Days later, my phone rang.

"Baby, I love you. Please don't be mad."

My heart dropped.

The car had been parked, and someone hit it. The damage was around $8,000. I was furious. I had no money left. I had already exhausted everything my father had left me. A few hundred dollars here and there wasn't enough. I was completely broke, but somehow, I still found a way to get the car fixed.

When he finally came back to Chicago, he pulled up high, laughing like everything was funny. I dropped him and his cousin off, and somehow, that turned into another huge argument. He jumped on me. He was a big man, about 6'8", 350 pounds. I'm 5'3". It got so bad that his cousins had to lock me in a room to separate us.

Then he went outside and destroyed my car, kicking the mirrors off, punching it, raging.

That was it.

I was done.

I prayed to God to get me out of that situation and to never let me turn back, and I didn't.

But life didn't suddenly get easier.

My grandmother passed away in a nursing home, all alone. She was an amazing woman who did everything for everyone. Losing her like that, especially after losing my father just two years before, was the worst feeling ever. On top of that, my mom's health was declining, and my finances were a mess. I had an expensive car note, my work hours were cut due to poor work ethics, and I was trying to help my mom while renovating my grandmother's building, where we all lived. It felt like I was being smothered by everything at once.

The Recipe to Life

Everything was closing in on me.

I was overwhelmed. I was exhausted. I was buried.

I was feeling smothered.

Just like smothered chicken, covered, weighed down, barely able to breathe, life had everything piled on top of me, and I was struggling to survive under the weight of it.

Smothered Chicken

Ingredients

- Chicken (whichever pieces you prefer)
- 2 tablespoons vegetable oil
- 1 cup flour
- 8 chicken bouillon cubes
- 1 stick butter
- 3 tablespoons Soulè Secret Seasoning
- 2 tablespoons paprika (plus extra for browning)
- 1 teaspoon salt
- 1 teaspoon ground black pepper
- 1 green bell pepper, sliced
- 1 red bell pepper, sliced
- 1 white onion, sliced
- 1 packet chicken brown gravy mix
- 2 cups chicken broth

Instructions

1. Prep the Chicken

Rinse your chicken and pat it dry. Coat the chicken lightly with vegetable oil so the seasoning sticks.

2. Season & Flour

Season the chicken with salt, black pepper, Soulè Secret Seasoning, and paprika. Once seasoned, roll each wing in flour until fully coated.

3. Layer the Dish

Place the floured chicken into a baking dish, spreading them out evenly.

Add the sliced green bell pepper, red bell pepper, and onion over the chicken.

4. Add the Flavor

Slice the stick of butter and place pieces throughout the pan.

Scatter the chicken bouillon cubes evenly across the dish

Sprinkle the chicken brown gravy mix over the top, followed by a little extra paprika for color and browning.

5. Pour & Cover

Slowly pour the chicken broth into the pan, making sure it settles around the chicken. Cover the dish tightly with foil.

6. Bake

Bake at **375°F** for **1 hour total**.

• After **30 minutes**, remove the foil.

• Return to the oven uncovered for the remaining **30 minutes** to let the chicken brown and the gravy thicken.

7. Serve

Once the chicken is tender, smothered, and golden brown, remove it from the oven and let it rest for a few minutes. Spoon that gravy right over the top and serve it up.

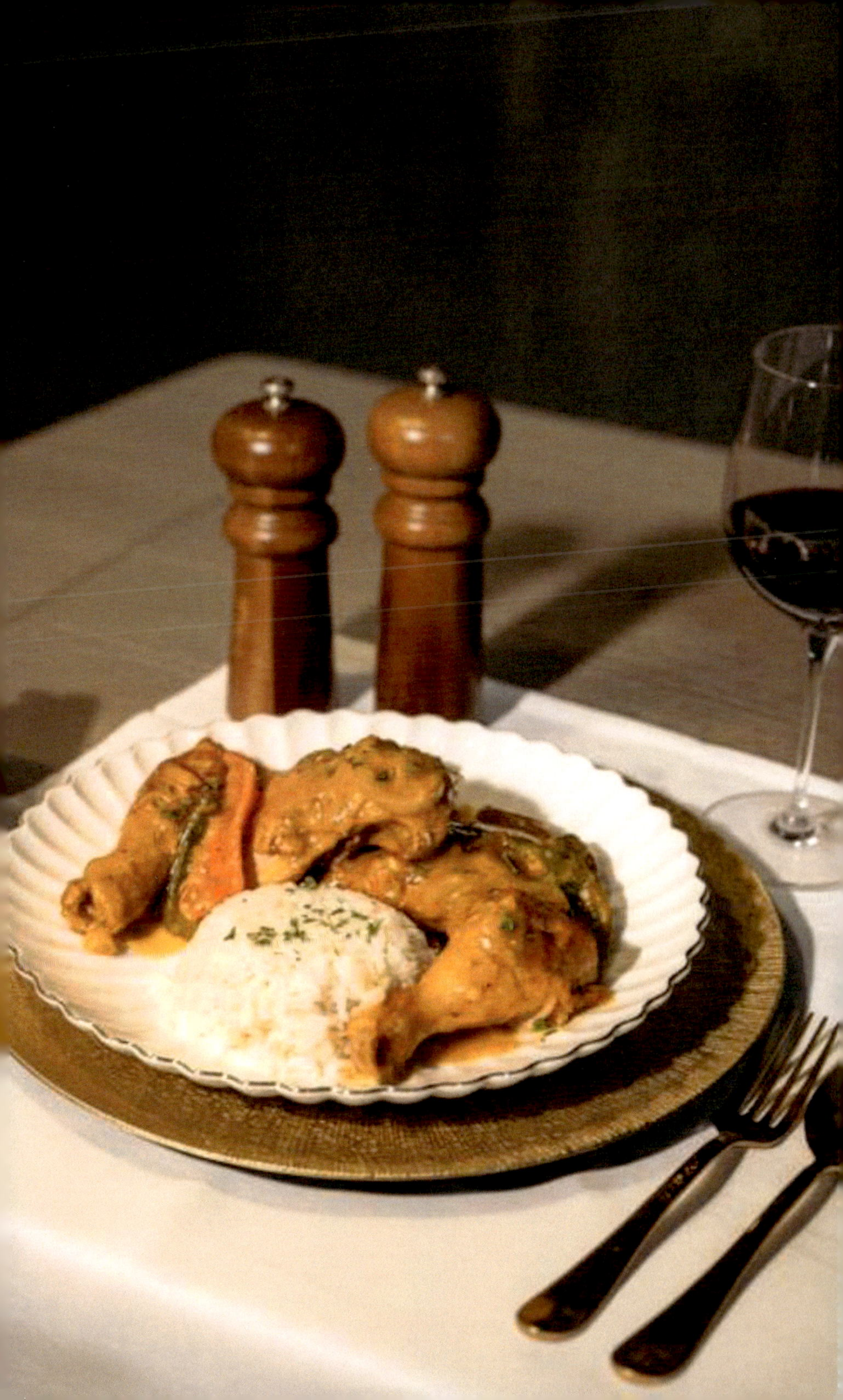

The Dirty Thirties – Dirty Rice

I went from having a man with me every single day to having nobody at all, and that shift hit me harder than I expected. I was already missing my dad and grandmother, already hurting, already broke. That little part-time Nike check wasn't doing nothing for me.

I needed a plan fast. I only knew one way to get it: back into the drug game. But I wasn't about to call him. I'd asked God to get me away from him, and I wasn't turning back.

It was one of those hot Chicago summer days, the kind where everybody's outside. My girls and I were on the Ave, Chicago Avenue on the West Side, where the block stays jumping. That's where I met B.

He was funny, dark, built right, and different from what I had just come from. We vibed instantly. He was a hustler, and for whatever reason, I was always drawn to that. We exchanged numbers, and just like that, he became my new man, or at least that's how he treated me.

But of course, just when I thought I had a good man, drama showed up.

One day, I pulled up and caught him arguing with a woman. I stayed in my car, watching, trying to figure out who the hell she was. When she pulled off, I finally asked him.

"That's my wife," he said.

My heart dropped straight into my stomach.

In my mind, I made excuses. I told myself they'd been married for only 30 days before we met. 30 days wasn't love, right? That marriage couldn't be real. I convinced myself he didn't love her like that. Foolish of me, but at the time, that lie helped me stay.

Every day after that, I was on the block with him. The block where he hustled was his territory. His grandmother owned a house on the block, and his whole family was around, including cousins, aunties, everybody. I'd be right there with them, sitting on the porch, watching my man hustle day in and day out. He had built that block. He was rolling. Money was coming in fast, and with that money came ego. And trust me, he started feeling *himself*… not *me*.

That's when I noticed the girls. Different ones pulling up all the time. My antennas were up. The block stayed packed, not just dope fiends, but women, too. His best friend was tall, fine, and a straight ladies' man, and together, they turned that block into a daily hangout.

Me and B started bumping heads heavy. He'd have me sitting on that porch while he stood on the block indulging these women he swore were "just friends."

B loved Remy. That was his drink. He'd drink it until he passed out. One night, he was laid out, knocked cold, and his phone would not stop ringing. I picked it up and didn't say a word. A woman was screaming on the other end, asking where he was and why he hadn't come fucked her. I finally spoke up and asked her who she was. She asked me the same. I told her straight: "I'm his girl."

I went back into the room and woke him up. "Get up. Right now." When he saw the phone in my hand, his face changed. I asked him who the bitch claiming him was. He snatched the phone, slapped me so hard, and told me to mind my business.

And just like that… the abuse started.

I found myself back in a hellhole. It was clear this man didn't give a damn about me. He was living his best life, and I was just there, feeling lonely. Then one day, me and my homegirl hit up this big annual boat party, the kind that's always lit, everybody shows up. After we get off the boat, I'm hungry, so we stop at a fast-food spot.

I'm standing in line when this guy bumps into me. I'm like, "Excuse you?" And he's all, "Damn, baby, my bad. You fine, though. Name's Tommy." I'm rolling my eyes like, "Who asked you?"

But I'll give it to him. Tommy was tall, dark, had that diamond watch, chain, dressed sharp, and had a nice smile. He even offered to buy me something to eat, telling me I was too uptight. And you know what? He made me laugh. He made me feel seen again.

He asked for my number. I hesitated because I knew B would lose it. Hell, he might even beat my ass. But I've always had a thing for playing with fire, so I gave it to him. And chileeee, I had no idea what kind of ride I was in for. Tommy was charming, flashy, full of it, and definitely a hustler, too.

We went full throttle. He wined and dined me, always had cash on him. I didn't ask how he got it; it was not my business. He knew about B, but he said he didn't care. That was a lie. As soon as we got intimate, he caught feelings and wanted me to leave B. Meanwhile, B was too busy with his new lifestyle to even notice I was slipping away.

Eventually, B and I had a blowout argument, and I told him I needed a break. Just like that, he ran back to his wife. I was sad, but I had Tommy, so I thought I'd be fine.

But a month in, I found out I was ten weeks pregnant. I was devastated. My baby's father was back with his wife, and I didn't want to get an abortion. I didn't want to let Tommy go either.

One day, I drove out to where Tommy was from to pick him up, and I could tell right away something was off. He was furious, pacing back and forth on the block with his people, talking fast, hands moving, energy heavy. When he finally got in the car, I found out he'd gotten into it with some of his own people. Things weren't good.

He was at war.

And when you're at war, hustling stops. Now it's about survival. That pocket full of money he used to flex? It was drying up fast. I started seeing the real picture: guns everywhere, paranoia, constant movement. Baby, I was not cut from that life. At all.

I was working here and there, but truth be told, the money I was getting from men was helping me keep my bills paid. Now he was broke, and I was panicking. On top of all that, I was pregnant, and neither Tommy nor B knew. I was a big girl, 289 pounds to be exact, but I wore it well. I knew how to dress, how to carry myself, how to hide what I needed to hide.

I knew Tommy was a hustler. What I didn't know was that he was a robber.

One day, I'm sitting in the car with Tommy and his cousin, and they're talking about a robbery, plotting it right in front of me like I wasn't even there. Not a kick-door type robbery, but a run-off. Taking people's money and drugs and disappearing. And the crazy part? It reminded me of how I'd been done before, how somebody just ran off with my stuff and left me empty.

Then Tommy tells me to meet him to eat. He invites another guy, and we're all sitting at the table, laughing, talking, breaking bread like everything is normal. I had no idea that man was his next victim.

Tommy had been down bad for a while. He had no

money and was stressed out. Then one day, he pops up at my house with his pockets full again. In my gut, I knew something wasn't right. I didn't ask where the money came from. I asked no questions.

A few days later, I'm by myself walking into the beauty supply when I see that same guy we had dinner with. Before I could even react, he grabbed me and said, "Where's Tommy?"

Something clicked instantly. I knew Tommy had done something foul to this man. I told him I didn't know where he was, that I hadn't seen him since dinner, that I'd been calling his phone. I even told him, "He probably with his woman. You'll see his bitch ass before I do."

I asked him what was wrong. He said, "Don't worry about it," and walked off.

In that moment, I thanked God. Because whatever Tommy did, that man could've taken it out on me, and he didn't. Right then and there, I knew I had to get away from Tommy's ass. No more playing with fire. This wasn't excitement anymore. This was danger.

I started finding every excuse not to deal with Tommy. I stopped answering his calls, stopped responding to his texts, stopped showing up. But he wasn't letting go. He kept pushing, kept insisting on seeing me, dead set on taking me to dinner. The truth was, I didn't want to be anywhere near him. I was scared of him. I didn't like him anymore. I was pregnant, sick, exhausted, and mentally checked out. I wanted out.

We got into a huge argument, and that's when it happened. Tommy hit me in my mouth.

Now let me be clear: I can be a little feisty with my mouth, but never disrespectful enough to deserve that. That was the last straw. That hit gave me my escape. I told him exactly how I felt about physical abuse, and from that day on, I never saw Tommy again for years.

And just like that, I was back home, man-less, pregnant, and ashamed.

I finally told my mother I was pregnant. I was embarrassed. I was about to be a single parent, with a sick mother to take care of, and I felt like I had failed her.

Then I called B and told him I was pregnant. But he and his wife were living their perfect life; there was no room for me in it. He told me he'd help with the baby, but he had no intention of being with me. That news made me sick to my stomach.

I kept asking myself, *How am I supposed to do this alone?*

A baby on the way. A sick mother. No father.

I had two sisters I knew would have my back, but I was the baby girl. I knew better. I felt like a disappointment.

B would still sneak and see me. He'd give me money. He'd make sure I ate. But at the end of the day, he was still going home to his wife.

One particular day, I needed money, and I needed it now. He told me to wait, and I didn't want to hear that. I was furious. I wanted him. I wanted my baby's father. I wanted security. I was tired of being alone. I was angry at everything.

So I pulled up to his grandmother's house on the block. I saw his car and told him to come outside. When he did, his wife came with him. She told me to leave. I refused. She walked up to my car and grabbed my door handle. I warned her, "Touch my car again, and I'm going to beat your ass."

She touched it again.

I got out and punched her.

Let me remind you, I was seven months pregnant.

B ran up and threw me to the ground for hitting his wife. That day turned into pure hell. Later on, I started cramping and ended up in the hospital, terrified I was losing my baby. B and his friends came to sit with me. Thank God, the baby was fine.

When we left, B was in the backseat with me. We started arguing again, and suddenly, he grabbed me by my neck. I jumped out of the car. He and his friend chased me down the street and forced me back inside the car. I was screaming, fighting, kicking, full of rage, not just at him, but at myself and every bad decision I had made.

They drove me to my mother's house and tried to walk me inside. I made it up the steps, still furious. I turned around and kicked his friend down the stairs because I didn't want him touching me. In return, B punched me on the side of my head. Later, it turned into a black eye.

My mother came outside furious. She told me to get in the house.

"God, what is wrong with me?" I asked as I prayed. All I could think about was the reckless decisions I kept making over and over again. I was tired of myself, tired of the cycle. *"God, change me,"* was my prayer.

I had gotten my ass kicked all day by men I loved, by choices I made, and by a life that was spinning completely out of control.

In the end, everything I went through in that chapter of my life was like throwing a wild mix of ingredients into a pot and turning up the heat. It was messy, it was chaotic, and it was full of moments that tested me to my core.

Just like dirty rice, it took all those scraps of experience, the heat, the bitterness, the unexpected spices, and turned them into something I could live with, learn from, and eventually share.

Now, let's take all that flavor and stir it into a pot, because this dirty rice recipe isn't just about food. It's about taking everything life threw at me and making it something you can taste.

Dirty Rice Recipe

Ingredients

- 1 lb. ground turkey
- 1 medium green bell pepper
- 1 medium red bell pepper
- 2 fresh jalapeños
- 1 small yellow onion, finely chopped
- 2 stalks celery, finely chopped
- 4 cloves garlic, finely chopped
- 1 tablespoon Creole seasoning
- 1 tablespoon Cajun seasoning
- 2 tablespoons cumin
- 1 cup Worcestershire sauce
- 3 tablespoons Louisiana hot sauce
- 2 tablespoons Soulè secret seasoning
- 3 tablespoons paprika
- 4 cups jasmine rice
- 4 cups chicken broth

- 1 teaspoon salt
- 1 teaspoon pepper

Instructions

1. Cook the Ground Turkey

In a nonstick skillet, add a splash of water and place the ground turkey in the skillet.

Season with cumin, paprika, Soulè secret seasoning, salt, and pepper.

Add about 1/2 cup of Worcestershire sauce for depth of flavor and color.

Continue to cook, chopping and stirring the meat until it's browned and cooked through.

2. Prepare the Rice:

In a separate pot, pour in the chicken broth and bring it to a boil.

Add the jasmine rice, chopped bell peppers, onions, jalapeños, and garlic. Stir well.

3. Combine and Simmer:

Once the rice and vegetables have started to cook, add the cooked ground turkey to the pot.

Pour in the remaining Worcestershire sauce, hot sauce,

Creole seasoning, and Cajun seasoning. Stir everything together thoroughly.

4. Cook to Perfection:

Let the mixture simmer for about 25 minutes, allowing the flavors to meld and the rice to become tender. Stir occasionally to ensure even cooking.

5. Serve:

Once everything is cooked and the rice is fluffy, remove from the heat.

Give it a final taste and adjust any seasonings as needed. Your dirty rice is ready to serve!

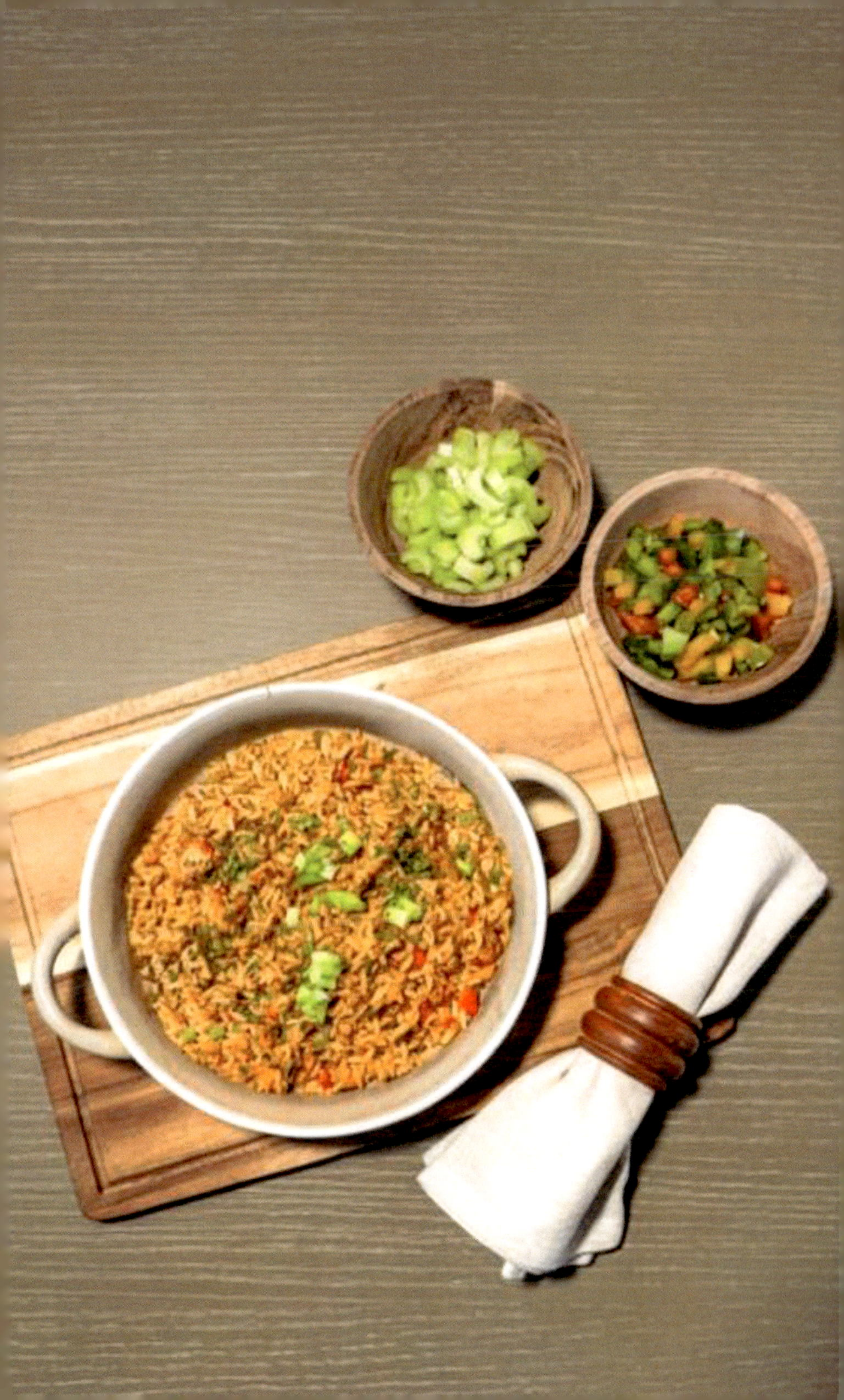

Getting to the Money – Mixed Greens with Smoked Turkey

Being pregnant and doing it all by myself was a fool. There was only so much I could do financially, and I was suffering. I was sick with my son, so sick I could barely eat. Everything made me nauseous. I was damn near bedridden, and working consistently wasn't even an option. My body just wouldn't allow it.

I'd look around and see everybody else living. My girls were outside. Gucci this, Louis that, cars, bags, trips. And me? I felt like I was damn near eating out of the garbage compared to how they were living. I was back in my mama's house, car on the repo list, pockets hurting, pride bruised. Baby, I needed in.

I started hanging around a few new girls, and when I tell you they had it going on, they had it going on. Clothes, bags, men with money, nice cars, their own cribs. I finally asked one of my homegirls to put me on. "How are y'all really getting money?" They told me all I needed was the people, and they'd make it happen. So, I got the people… but nothing happened.

I sat back and watched them make cash money while I stayed stuck. And believe it or not, it just didn't work for me the way it worked for them. But what did work was when I moved on my own.

I've always been a hustler. I sit back, I watch, I ask questions. I've never been afraid to use my resources. That's when I ended up meeting one of B's cousins. We were just talking, nothing heavy at first. Then I realized she was in the same game as the girls I'd been hanging with.

But this was different.

She was cool as hell. Gangster. An ultimate hustler. People did not play with her. She didn't mind carrying a gun, and she damn sure wasn't scared to use it if it came down to it. She didn't gatekeep. She taught me the game I had been asking to learn. She gave me everything I needed to know, the real rules, the real moves, the kind of knowledge that was about to put me on the map.

All she had to do was show me one time, and after that, it was on and popping. I was getting into the money, real money. I was making more than the very friends who were supposed to put me on in the first place. Funny how that works. Next thing you know, *they* needed *me*.

And because I'm not a gatekeeper, I showed them the game, too. I couldn't get all the money by myself anyway, no matter how much they felt like I could. My name started ringing. Word spread. Now I had more "friends" in the same game, or at least I thought they were friends. Truth was, a lot of people just wanted to be around to see what I had going on. Because in this life, what's hot today can be gone tomorrow.

That's when I started doing business with this new girl. And baby, she had a bag bag. Big money. We got close, almost like besties. She was a hustling-ass chick with all the bells and whistles: nice crib, nice car, and every designer bag you could think of. Me and her were running it up together. We were everywhere: BET Awards, clubs, money flowing, living fast. Believe it or not, we were rolling.

But even with all that money coming in, something didn't sit right with me. I knew, deep down, God wasn't going to bless no mess. I knew I wasn't raised like this. And in that moment, I had to admit the truth: I had become a product of my environment.

That's when I made a decision. I said, I want to turn this into something legitimate. And that's exactly what I did.

Before I get into opening my business office, me and B found our way back to each other. Somehow, we started vibing again. He left his wife, and just like that, we became a family. The weight of being a single parent was lifted off my shoulders. I gave birth to a beautiful baby boy, weighing 7 pounds 11 ounces, on 7/7/2007. How lucky was he?

Life felt different then. I was still hustling, but truth be told, I was out-hustling B. I had the plan. I had the vision. Eventually, we moved in together, and in the middle of all that motion, I rediscovered something I loved: doing hair. I'd be over at B's grandmother's house practicing styles on his family, getting my hands back into it. It took me back to my Jackson State days, when I was doing hair and eyebrows nonstop. Five-dollar flips, three-dollar brows, line out the door; I was hustling even back then.

I loved his family, and they loved my baby and me. I ended up spending more time at their house than my own mama's. My mother was dealing with serious health issues, even though at the time, I told myself she was doing better. She wasn't. She had a rare muscle deterioration disease, one in five million, along with lupus and other autoimmune issues. Her body was failing her.

I'd go upstairs, clean her, bathe her, feed her. She had a caregiver, Junior, who helped, too, but some days were just hard. Watching a woman who once lived so fully become bedridden was heartbreaking. She cried often, feeling forgotten, like life had moved on without her. Now that I'm older, I understand her pain. People don't always leave intentionally; life just keeps moving.

At times, hustling felt so good. I was everywhere, parties, popping bottles, custom clothes being made, buying bags, nice car, in and out of town. As people would say, I was *popping my shit.* The world felt like it was mine. I didn't need for nothing.

My mama was straight, at least from the outside. She knew I was up to something, but what I was doing felt like the least of our worries compared to the disease she was fighting, the one that completely changed her life.

The way I was getting money blinded me to the steady

decline of my mother's health. I was running the streets left and right, chasing a high that felt unstoppable. At one point, I had saved over $100,000, and back in the early 2000s, that was big. I was far from humble. I was in my glo. And like they say, being a Gemini comes with two sides: one side telling me to keep hustling, the other whispering that it was time to get on a straight and narrow path.

In the middle of all that, something else started growing. While practicing hairstyles on my baby father's family, I started getting good, really good. Just being me, doing what I liked, I found myself working in a shop without a license. I thought I had a small clientele at first, but it didn't stay small for long. Word spread. Chair stayed full.

I had a lot on my plate: a new baby, a sick mother, money still coming in from the streets, and now I was a hairstylist, too. But no matter how much I hustled or how deep I got in the streets, I always knew I wanted a positive life for myself. My mother and father may have lived that life, but they didn't raise me to stay in it. They wanted better for my sisters and me.

So I kept looking for the right way to do things. I went back to school, not Jackson State this time, but Paul Mitchell Hair School. Outside of my love for money, I genuinely loved styling hair. It gave me peace. Purpose.

I started shying away from hustling. I had saved enough. I was ready to turn things around. I was on a positive track, hair school, goals, vision. That's when I opened up my business office, and baby, I was booming. My name was ringing everywhere. I knew how to help people get maximum money fast. I had so much coming in that I was even lending money, waiting on people to flip what I put in for them.

I was helping people get on, but not too much, because I knew my end goal. I wanted out. I wanted to be 100% legitimate. In the meantime, in between times, I had over 300 clients. When I say I was rolling, I was rolling. And of course, with rolling comes hate. Some people felt a way. Some people were only around for the wrong reasons. I didn't care at the time; all I could see was the money. My phone rang day in and day out.

I still had money in the streets, but most of my income was coming from my office. I was transitioning. When that season ended, my hair business took off even more. I was damn near out the game. My plan was clear: to be a popular hairstylist, a business owner, and a provider. I wanted to give my son a great life, and my family, too.

Dear God,

Thank You for covering me. Please order my steps.

You've been giving me grace my entire life, even when I didn't always deserve it.

Please continue to keep Your hand on me.

This was the prayer I prayed when I was trying to find my way out of the streets and into a better life. I didn't have all the answers; I just knew I needed Him to lead me.

In the end, I realized that all the hustling, all the lessons, and all the love for creating something of my own was like cooking a pot of mixed greens. It was about taking what I had, my roots, my resilience, my determination, and turning it into something real and nourishing. Just like those greens, you let them simmer with smoked turkey, and it becomes a dish full of flavor and soul, just like the life I was building.

So let's get into the kitchen and turn all that hustle and heart into a pot of mixed greens with smoked turkey. This is more than just a recipe; it's a taste of the journey.

Mixed Greens

Ingredients

- 4 smoked turkey tails
- ½ cup vegetable oil
- 4 bushels collard greens
- 4 bushels mustard greens
- 4 bushels turnip greens
- 1 yellow onion, diced
- ½ cup Soulè Secret Seasoning
- 2 pepperoncino peppers
- 2 tablespoons vinegar
- 1 teaspoon salt
- 1 tablespoon black pepper
- 3 tablespoons chicken soup base
- 1 teaspoon sugar
- 2 cups chicken broth

Instructions

1. Boil the Meat

In a large stock pot, add the smoked turkey tails and cover with water.

Boil until the meat is tender, and the broth is rich and flavorful.

2. Prep the Greens

While the turkey tails are cooking, wash the greens **very well**; you already know, greens hold dirt.

Roll the greens into tight bundles and slice them.

3. Braise the Greens

In a large sauté pan, add the chicken broth and diced onions.

Sauté until the onions are soft and fragrant.

Add the sliced greens and braise them until they begin to wilt and soften.

4. Bring It Together

Transfer the braised greens and onions into the stock pot with the turkey tails.

Add:

- Vinegar
- Pepperoncino peppers

- Sugar (to cut the bitterness)

- Vegetable oil (this helps break the greens down)

- Salt, pepper, chicken soup base, and Soulè Secret Seasoning

5. Simmer Low & Slow

Cover the pot and let the greens cook on medium-low heat for **about 1½ hours**, stirring occasionally.

6. Taste & Adjust

Now listen, ladies and gentlemen… we come from households where **we don't measure**.

Taste as you go and adjust the seasoning to **your preference** until it's just right.

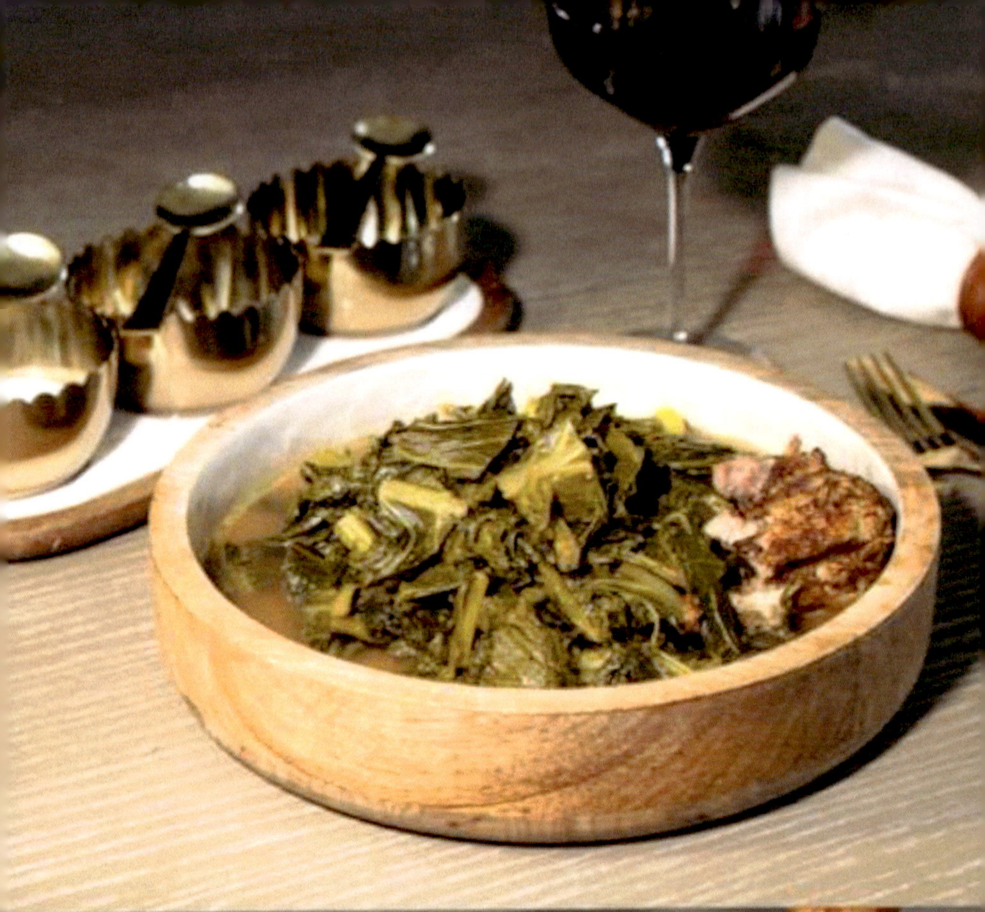

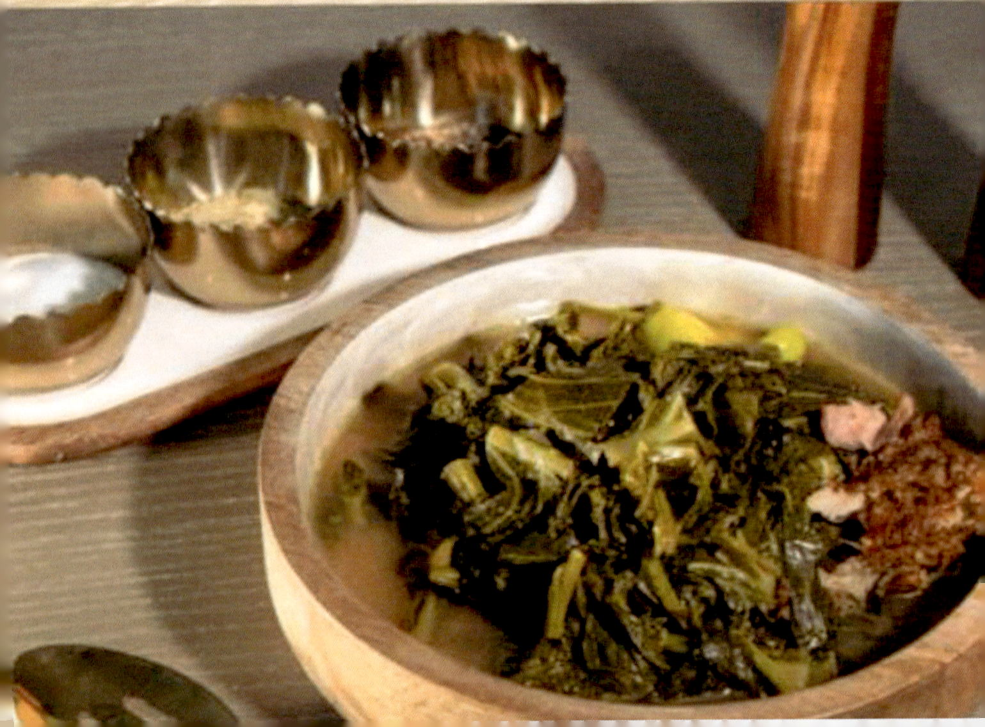

Thinking Shit Sweet – Sweet Potatoes

Life was going great as far as money went, but me and B? We were just cool. And by cool, I mean he was still a ladies' man, and I was letting a lot of shit slide. I was getting so much money that I wasn't even paying his ass no attention. I was just happy to have him around, helping with our son. But B did whatever he wanted to do, and infidelity stayed being a headache. Women after women. Constant disrespect. And somehow, I kept putting up with it.

The abuse didn't stop either. If anything, it got worse.

But in the midst of all that, there were these moments of stillness, like the day I stayed home. Anyone who knows me knows I love music. Back then, I'd sit around downloading songs, making CDs. I'm not sure why I stayed in that day. Usually, I'd be out running the streets, collecting money, living day to day. But that day was different.

I could barely boil water; I never knew how to cook much, but sometimes my mom and I would cook together. Her home care provider would put her in her wheelchair, and she'd sit in the kitchen, telling me step by step how to make a dish.

I called her from downstairs. B and I lived in the basement. I said, "Mom, have Junior put you in your wheelchair and let's make some short ribs." But she told me she didn't feel well. She was on the phone with her sisters, calling everyone, saying she wasn't feeling right. The night before, I'd given her some Chinese food with MSG by mistake, and I thought maybe that's why she felt off.

I stood in the kitchen, looking down the hall, joking, "Girl, you need to take your ass to the doctor." She just kept talking on the phone. I got in the tub, still half-laughing, thinking she was just calling for help like she sometimes did when nothing was really wrong. But then her home care provider knocked on the bathroom door and told me to come help. I wrapped a towel around me, ran to her side, and asked, "Mom, are you okay?" She shook her head no.

I called 911, ran to my uncle upstairs, and begged him to come help. He and my mom hadn't talked for months, but he came down. He tried to snap her out of it, but she didn't respond. He looked at me, and I could see he knew. I was screaming, panicking, calling my sisters, yelling for help from the neighbors. We were all like family on that block.

They took her out on a stretcher and worked on her right there. She always said if the sirens were on, you'd be fine. They left with the sirens on, so I thought we had time. I thought she would be fine. I got dressed slowly, thinking she'd be okay.

When I got to the hospital, my sister was laying on the ground of the parking lot, crying. She told me Mom didn't make it. I couldn't believe it. I thought I had time. But that was it. My mother was gone. Me asking her if she was okay was the last time I would communicate with my mother.

The Recipe to Life

My mother's death didn't feel real at all. I didn't know how to process it, so I did what I'd always done with loss: I ran. Just like with my father and my grandmother, I stayed busy and convinced myself she was just on vacation somewhere, that she'd be back. Facing the truth felt impossible.

When it came time to bury her, I was in charge of making sure she looked exactly like herself. My mother loved her sideburns, and I used to tease her, telling her that when she passed, I was going to cut them off. It was our little joke. I never imagined I'd actually be standing there, scissors in hand, preparing her for her final rest.

Walking into that room and seeing my mother's lifeless body on the table nearly took me out. I almost passed out. She didn't look like herself at all; she was pale, almost blue. I remember asking the funeral director who that woman was, because in that moment, I couldn't accept that it was my mom. They explained the process, the massage cream that had to be used before makeup could be applied, but none of it mattered. The woman lying there didn't resemble the mother I knew, my light-skinned, beautiful mom.

When I finally found the courage, her best friend and I began working on her together. Her best friend painted her nails: *Forever Red*, her favorite color. I cut and styled her hair and, of course, I left her sideburns just the way she loved them. I did her makeup, too. She loved Fashion Fair, and I made sure her face reflected that love and care.

When I finished, I finally recognized the woman lying on that table. It was my mother. She was beautiful again. I talked to her as if she were still alive, and that's how I made it through: by pretending she could still hear me. Red was her favorite color, so we dressed her in a red suit and sent her home to glory.

After the funeral, I went back to running, running from death, from my past, and from the reality I wasn't ready to face.

I went from being on the block every day to barely being there at all because I was hustling so heavy. One day, I decided to pull back up, just to check the scene. And baby… it was a lot going on. B had this new "worker," and I felt it in my spirit immediately: something wasn't right. He swore she was just there to help, but she walked that block like she owned it. In his car every day. Loud. Bold. And she made it her mission to get under my skin every time she saw me.

One day, I wasn't having the best day. I was in my feelings, tired, not looking my best. I pulled up to pick up my son from B's grandmother's house and heard her on the porch next door with some of his other workers. She was pointing me out, telling the new girl, "That's B's baby mama." Then I heard somebody say B was bogus, like I wasn't that girl.

I turned around with my baby in my arms and asked them who the fuck they thought they were playing with.

Words were exchanged, and I told them straight, "I'd

be back." I had my baby with me, so I wasn't fighting right then. I called my sister immediately. Everybody knows the middle one does not play. I'm not a fighter, but my sister? She's a force.

I dropped my baby off with my neighbor, picked my sister up, and we went right back to the block. By the time we pulled up, the whole block was packed. She had her sister with her as well it was a straight showdown. We started arguing, and one of B's friends tried to stand between us. In my mind, I was the queen bee. Nobody should've even let her touch me.

But I was angry. Full of rage.

I smacked her.

Then I smacked her again.

The third time, his friend stepped out of the way, and we fought.

That was the longest fight of my life. I didn't lose, but I didn't feel like I won either. My sister damn near beat the other sister unconscious. The whole block had to break it up. And when it was over, the truth finally came out: B was messing with her.

I lost again, not because of her, but because I should've walked away. She wasn't worth it. I stooped low. I hated B for putting me there.

I kept doing hair, but my office was seasonal, and the

money started slowing down again. That's when one of my homeboys called me and told me he had a lick–the newest scam. I didn't want to go back down that road, but baby, this shit looked sweet. Watching him get material things damn near for free had me curious. You mean all I gotta do is walk in the store, grab what I want, and walk out?

Put me on or leave me alone.

And he put me on.

I was back in the game, but a different kind of hustle. Looking back now, only God was covering me, because I wouldn't dare have the courage to do half that shit today. I was getting so much merch and meeting people all over, from the South Side to the West Side. I was moving.

Then, one night, I'm at a party, and guess who I see?

Tommy.

He looked good, like he always did. Bells and whistles. Life looked sweet on him, too. B and I were on bad terms, so was it hard for Tommy to get my attention again? Not at all. How could I keep doing this to myself? But baby… the flesh wants what the flesh wants.

Tommy seemed different this time, or so I thought. He was nicer. Calmer. It felt like he had done a whole 360. I'd be out hustling, and he didn't mind. He stayed right by my side, never asking for nothing, just protecting me while I was out throwing rocks at the penitentiary.

Tommy and I became cool. Not every day, but when I had free time, I'd pull up to his block, and we'd hang out. Everybody knew me over there. He became my peace. Crazy how somebody you once hated can turn into your best friend, right?

With B, it wasn't just physical abuse; it was mental, too. Sundays were supposed to be our family day. Dinner, movies, just us. That was my one day a week. And then that stopped, too. I did everything B wanted. Had his back through all the cheating. When those Sundays disappeared, I knew we were done.

One day, I asked him, "What about family day? What about me?"

He looked at me and said I didn't even deserve that.

That crushed me.

I knew his time was up.

The farther I got from B, the closer I got back to Tommy. Five years went by, and I ended up back with him. I washed B's clothes, dropped them off at his mama's house, gave him thousands of dollars, and walked away. That was my care package. I wasn't petty; I was done.

I know y'all thinking, What the hell were you thinking?

Same shit I'm thinking today. I'm with y'all.

Tommy was by my side every day then. He was on house arrest, but I didn't ask too many questions. I knew he had been in trouble. Some nights we talked, some nights we didn't. I asked if he was dating. He said he had a "friend."

Chileeee.

That "friend" was actually the woman whose house he was on house arrest at. When I found that out, I was furious. So mad I bonded him off house arrest. Five thousand dollars. Nothing to me. I could make that in a day.

Now he was all mine. Or so I thought.

I had the money. He had the block. It felt right to put him on. I believe you help people you care about, and that's exactly what I did. Not because I had to.

But because I thought shit was sweet.

I invested in Tommy so he could get his block rolling again. Things started looking up for him. And let me tell you, Tommy already knew how to look good, but with me by his side and the things I was doing, baby, he was living like a king. I had just bought a new Jaguar, baby Jaguar, and it stood out everywhere. Sometimes he'd drive it, soaking it all in. He was living his best life, really his best lie, with me.

One night at dinner, Tommy asked me for some money, and I was confused. Confused because I had already given him money to start his business, and from the outside, the block looked like it was doing well.

“So where’s your re-up money?” I asked.

He told me his last order wasn’t right and that he couldn’t get his money back. And because I felt bad and I had money lying around, I gave him what he asked for. Meanwhile, I was hustling nonstop, still doing hair, juggling everything. My life was all over the place.

Tommy would go hours without answering his phone. Now, if you’ve ever dealt with a street guy, you know that can happen. But his “busy” wasn’t the right kind of busy. He was busy with that “friend” of his. I started getting private calls. People from the streets were telling me he was playing me. I didn’t want to hear it.

I threw Tommy a birthday party, spent a bag on it. His friends were there, the vibes were up. And when we walked out the door… there she was. The “friend.” She knocked his ass out cold. Right then and there, everything was confirmed. That “friend” wasn’t just a friend; she was the woman he was dealing with. The woman he was actually in love with.

My heart broke.

I later found out the truth: the whole time, Tommy was just paying me back, swindling me, buttering me up, because he wanted his get-back. He told me when I left him years ago, I broke his heart. He thought I left because he didn’t have money. That wasn’t true. I left because he was living recklessly, and I didn’t want that life.

Even knowing the truth, I let him keep finding his way back in. One week he'd be with her, the next week with me. Blowout after blowout. Then he came to me again for the third time, asking for re-up money. I couldn't understand it.

"How do you not have money again?"

This time, it was a hard no.

That's when I found out he was taking care of her.

He later told me he never really did anything for me because I already had everything. And I told him straight, "Bitch, Beyoncé got everything. You think Jay-Z wouldn't buy her anything because she got it all?" That's when I knew: this man had me fucked up.

One of the times I took him back, the girl called my phone. She told me Tommy had jumped on her. I didn't believe it. I was on the phone defending him, telling her he'd never do that, like I had amnesia about him hitting me in the mouth years ago.

Until it was my turn.

I can't even remember what triggered it. Maybe she had broken up with him. Maybe it was his frustration. But things went left, and he jumped on me. I was done. I couldn't believe it. How did I end up back here? This was the third man to put his hands on me.

That's when I knew: this shit was out of control.

I stopped dealing with Tommy. In between that time, I met another guy. He was sweet, but honestly, I was just done with men altogether. We talked here and there, nothing serious.

But somehow… my slow ass let Tommy back in.

For the third time.

Dear Lord,

I know they say You look out for babies and fools.

I was the fool You always looked over.

Please continue to have mercy on me and on the bad decisions I made.

Those decisions came from hurt and pain, not from who I truly am.

Thank You for never giving up on me, even when I didn't know how to choose myself.

In the end, I had to realize I'd been tasting a kind of sweetness that wasn't real. Life can be a lot like a pot of candied yams, full of sugar, full of spice, and everything nice stirred together in one pot. But just like that dish, you have to simmer through the tough moments to find the real flavor.

Candied Sweet Potatoes (Soulè-Style)

Ingredients

- 8–10 sweet potatoes, peeled and sliced
- 2 cups water
- 1 cup of imitation vanilla extract
- 2 sticks butter
- 1 tablespoon cinnamon
- 1 tablespoon nutmeg
- 2 cups granulated sugar
- 1 cup brown sugar

Instructions

This recipe is pretty simple; no extra steps, no fancy tricks.

1. Prep the Sweet Potatoes

Rinse, peel, and slice the sweet potatoes.

Once cleaned, place them into a large stock pot.

2. Build the Flavor

Pour in the water, then season the potatoes with:

- Cinnamon
- Nutmeg
- Granulated sugar
- Brown sugar

Place the butter right on top, then pour in the **imitation vanilla**.

3. Cook Them Down

Cover the pot, turn the heat to **medium**, and let everything come to a boil.

4. Adjust the Syrup (Optional)

If you like a **thicker syrup**, remove the lid after about **30 minutes** and let the sweet potatoes simmer uncovered for another **15 minutes**, stirring occasionally.

5. Servc

Once tender and glossy, they're ready.

Soft, sweet, and cooked all the way through, just how they're supposed to be.

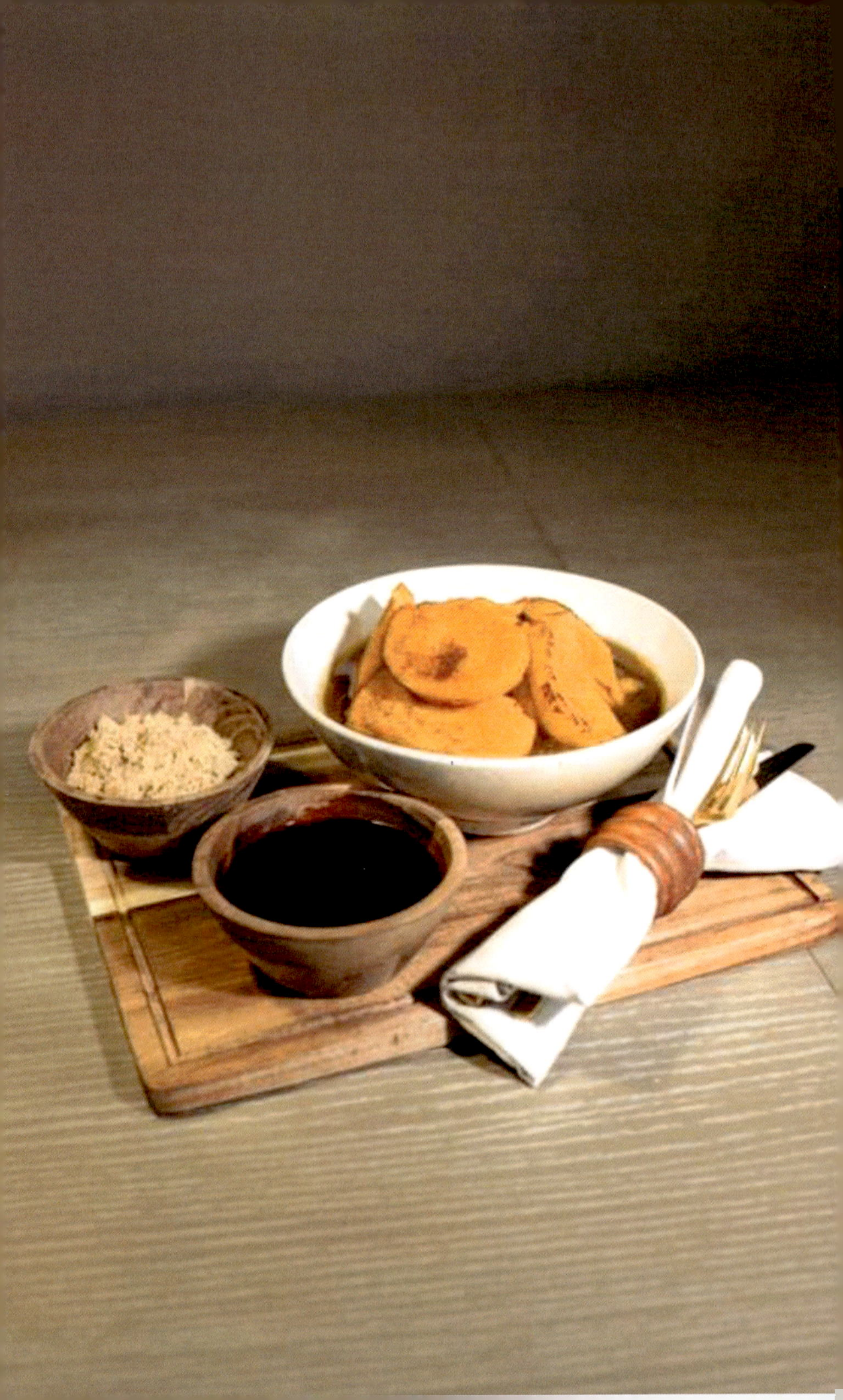

The Meltdown – Mac and Cheese

Tommy came back crying and apologizing, but I meant what I said. Three strikes, you're out. And this time, I stood on it.

If I'm being honest, taking Tommy back felt like I was competing with the other girl more than fighting for the relationship. I think I had checked out emotionally a long time ago, but I hated the idea of losing. This was one battle I finally surrendered. I was tired.

Earlier that day, Tommy picked me up from work, and I dropped him off on the block. After that, I went and picked up my homegirl, someone I looked up to like a big sister. She was what we called the *big homie*. She had her life together and didn't play about men, money, cars, clothes, or life, period. Riding around with her, I opened up about everything I'd been carrying: Tommy, my mom passing, the weight of it all. I had a lot going on.

As I mentioned in a previous chapter, I had met someone new. His name was Sur. He was calm, laid-back, and genuinely kind. We talked on the phone here and there, nothing heavy. That day, we had plans to hang out. But while I was waiting on Sur to link up with me, something didn't sit right. Tommy had been too quiet for too long.

I called his phone. No answer.

So I did what my intuition told me to do: I went to his block.

I pulled up and saw all his friends, but not him. I started asking around, "Where's Tommy? Where's Tommy?" Everyone looked at me like I was crazy, like they didn't know me. Something felt off. Real off.

As I drove away, I caught a glimpse out of the corner of my eye: Tommy's hat. I backed the car up. There he was, sitting on the curb… with *her*. The same girl he promised he wasn't dealing with anymore. The same girl who looked me in my face and said they were done.

I rolled down the window and asked, "So this is what we're doing?"

He looked at me with pure rage, biting his bottom lip. She sat there, enjoying every second of it, front-row seat to my heartbreak.

We went back and forth, arguing. My homegirl got out of the car and came to the driver's side when she saw how upset I was. She told me to stay calm, but I was already past that point.

I looked at him and said, "Fuck all this. What are you about to do? Are you coming with me, or are you staying here with her?"

And he chose her.

That was the worst mistake of his life.

You never choose anyone over me.

From that day on, I never spoke to Tommy again. He called over and over, but there was no answer. Sent friends to reach out, still nothing. Slowly, he started to fade. He didn't look the same anymore. His glow was gone. The water was cut off, literally and figuratively. He had been living his best life, and I was the one helping support it.

That day marked the end of Tommy's era in my life.

The meltdown was real, but sometimes, things have to fall apart completely before you can finally walk away for good.

When I left Tommy's block, Sur and I went on our first real date, and from that day on, we were together.

Life with Sur was completely different. He was laid-back, patient, and kind. He treated me well, and he was good to my son. He felt like a breath of fresh air. I was still carrying so much pain from my past: toxic relationships, losing my mother, all of it. But Sur never judged me. Not once. He felt heaven-sent.

We started dating nonstop. I smiled every day, *all day*. Sur bought me cards and flowers at least twice a week. I had never experienced that kind of intentional love before. He gave thoughtful, nice gifts, but more than that, he was just… nice. I was finally at peace. Everything felt perfect.

Meanwhile, Tommy was still calling and making threats. He wasn't in a good place mentally, and I ignored him, thinking it was all talk.

Until it wasn't.

One day, Sur dropped me off at home. I walked in on a high; you know that beginning stage when it's all butterflies and excitement, when everything feels new and fun. But the moment I stepped inside, something felt wrong. The energy was off.

I called one of my homegirls and stayed on the phone, just so I wouldn't be alone. We were talking, but deep down, I could *feel* someone else in the house. I can't explain it; just a presence.

Before I could even process it, Tommy came from under my bed. He had a knife. He was sweating. Angry. And I was terrified.

I tried to calm him down while secretly texting my friend to call the police. All I could think was, *This man has lost his mind.* I kept asking him how he got into my house. He looked at me and said, "Anything man-made can be broken."

Then he said, "You think I'm a joke? You think you're just gonna live life with a new man and leave me behind?"

He told me to call Sur and tell him never to come back, that we were done.

I refused.

That's when he punched me in my face.

Then he pressed the knife against my side and said, "Call him. Now."

I called Sur. He answered, "What's up, baby?"

And with my heart breaking, I said, "Please don't ever come back over here. Don't call me again. Just forget about me."

He was confused and kept saying, "What?" but I hung up.

The police felt like they were taking forever. Tommy kept making threats, pacing, raging… and then he walked out the door. By the grace of God, he didn't kill me. He hurt me, but I was alive.

As he walked down the stairs, the police were coming up, and he got away.

I remember thinking, *Chile… what have I gotten myself into?* Just when I thought life was finally good, here comes this chaos.

I called Sur and explained everything. He already knew something was wrong; he knew we were vibing too hard, too real, for it to end like that. There was a lot of back and forth after that with Tommy and Sur. But one thing was certain:

I never heard from Tommy again.

I was still hustling, learning the *right* way to do the *wrong* things. Just when I thought I was changing my life, I was actually getting in deeper. But there's always a warning before destruction. God has a funny way of sending signs, and there were so many little things happening around me that made me want to get out of the game.

I still had my office business, which was 100% legit. I didn't play about that. But because I stopped being what I call a *financial magician*, I lost a lot of clients. I was no longer bending rules or making miracles happen. So once again, I had one foot in and one foot out.

My business was clean, but I was still dipping and dabbing in other things to make money, just being greedy. On the outside, everything looked fine. I had money, material things, and a nice car. I was even renovating my mom's house room by room. Life looked okay.

Then, one day, I got a call from a homeboy who was locked up. He told me investigators had come to see him about some business we had done *years* ago.

I was scared as shit.

Not long after that, a former client called me and said investigators had questioned them about something I'd done for them years back, the same type of situation my homeboy mentioned. That's when panic set in. I started watching everything and everyone around me. And if you know me, you know I'm already an overthinker.

Then some of the girls I used to hustle with started saying *they* were getting visits, too.

Baby… I felt like my whole life was tumbling down.

They were questioning people one by one, and I thought I was next. I was nervous, but the truth was, I hadn't been involved with that particular group or that hustle in a long time. Years. I wasn't doing it anymore. I knew there were statutes of limitation, but fear doesn't care about logic.

What if someone threw me under the bus?

At that point, all I could do was wait and see what God had in store for me.

Through all of this, Sur was my peace.

We did everything together, partied together, traveled together. We loved Atlanta. We'd go just to vibe. On one trip, we went to this soul food restaurant called *Busy Bee's*. Baby… those yeast rolls took me *out*.

They reminded me of my Grandma Bee. One bite, and it woke something up in me. Memories flooded back. I missed my family. My sisters and I had drifted apart, each doing our own thing, and I missed that closeness so much. I felt this strong urge to bring us back together.

It's crazy how eating a yeast roll made me want to open a restaurant.

Now, mind you, y'all know damn well I didn't know *anything* about the restaurant business. Hell, I barely knew how to boil water. But something about those yeast rolls did it for me. Those rolls were a blessing that helped change the direction of my life.

When we headed back to Chicago, all I could think about was what I was going to do next.

Not long after that, I woke up extremely sick. My stomach was cramping so bad, sharp pains I couldn't explain. Sur took me to the doctor.

I was pregnant.

Lord… what am I gonna do with a baby?

I cried day and night. I was scared of the investigators, scared of the unknown. I felt like I was just getting into my glow, just starting to live, just beginning something real with Sur, and now I had to share him with a baby. Selfish? Maybe. But it was real.

Sur was excited, though, and that helped.

If I'm being honest, I hated being pregnant. Just like with my first son, I was sick the entire time. I couldn't do hair. I barely hustled. I couldn't get out of bed. I was sick as hell.

On Valentine's Day, Sur wanted to go to Vegas. I was seven months pregnant and terrified to fly; I'd been told you shouldn't fly late in pregnancy, but I went anyway.

We made it to the hotel… and that's when it happened.

Sur proposed.

He wanted to get married *that day*. I said yes, but truthfully, I wasn't ready. Chileeee, my mind was everywhere. How could I not want to marry this man? He was perfect. But I was fighting so much internally.

I was depressed. Still grieving my mother, my father, my grandmother. Still worried about investigators. Still carrying fear that I hadn't spoken out loud.

I asked him to give me time.

I know I broke his heart.

We stayed in Vegas a few more days. I laid in that bed thinking… praying. And one morning I woke up and said, "Sur, let's get married."

He was so excited.

We went to the courthouse, did the paperwork, then walked into a small chapel and got married, right there in Las Vegas.

Sur never liked me hustling. Not at all. He didn't want that life for me, never did. He always said I deserved better, even when I didn't fully believe it myself.

When I finally had the baby, a beautiful baby girl, she became the apple of Sur's eye. He loved that baby like nothing I had ever seen. From the moment we found out I was pregnant, Sur never missed a single doctor's appointment. Not one. He was always right there, holding my hand, steady and proud.

He used to say she was his love child, and he bragged about her every chance he got. He was the first person she saw when she entered this world. She was perfect. Chunky, head full of hair, and special in a way I can't explain.

After she was born, I stopped doing hair. I stopped hustling. All I could think about was that restaurant, the one I knew I was going to open one day.

I started small, working on recipes, teaching myself how to cook. I made easy dishes at first: tacos. Once I mastered them, y'all know me… the hustle kicked back in. I started selling dollar tacos and five-dollar Patron snowballs. I was still finding ways to make money, just trying to survive.

For a while, life was calm. Everything felt okay.

Then I got the call.

The feds had come knocking at one of my girlfriend's doors. They had all the evidence they needed to build a case against her. My heart dropped. I just knew they were coming for me next.

All I could do was pray.

God, I want to change my life. I want to be better. Please, if You save me from whatever is coming my way, I promise I'll never disappoint You again. God, please give me this restaurant. This is my way out. Use my hands. Teach me how to prepare meals. I can't go to jail. My two kids need me. I'm not built for prison.

I prayed day and night.

And I came up with a plan.

I had a little money saved, not much, but I needed a way out for my kids and me. I always wanted to give them a better life than the one I had. I never wanted them to experience the pain, fear, or survival mode I had lived in for so long.

As strong as I had always been, everything inside me was melting down.

I felt weak.

I felt vulnerable.

I was scared.

I was depressed.

And for the first time in my life, I was willing to give up *everything* just for a chance at a new beginning.

The Recipe to Life

There was a time when it felt like everything in my life was melting down. One moment, I was in control, and the next, everything, my fear, my survival, my past, was bubbling over. I had to learn that when life is boiling hot, you either break apart or you transform. And trust me, I fought that transformation every step of the way. But sometimes, you realize that the heat is doing something. Slowly, things soften. They blend. They become something richer than they were before. In my life, I had to trust that the meltdown wasn't the end; it was just the start of something amazing.

Now let's get into this Mac and Cheese Recipe!

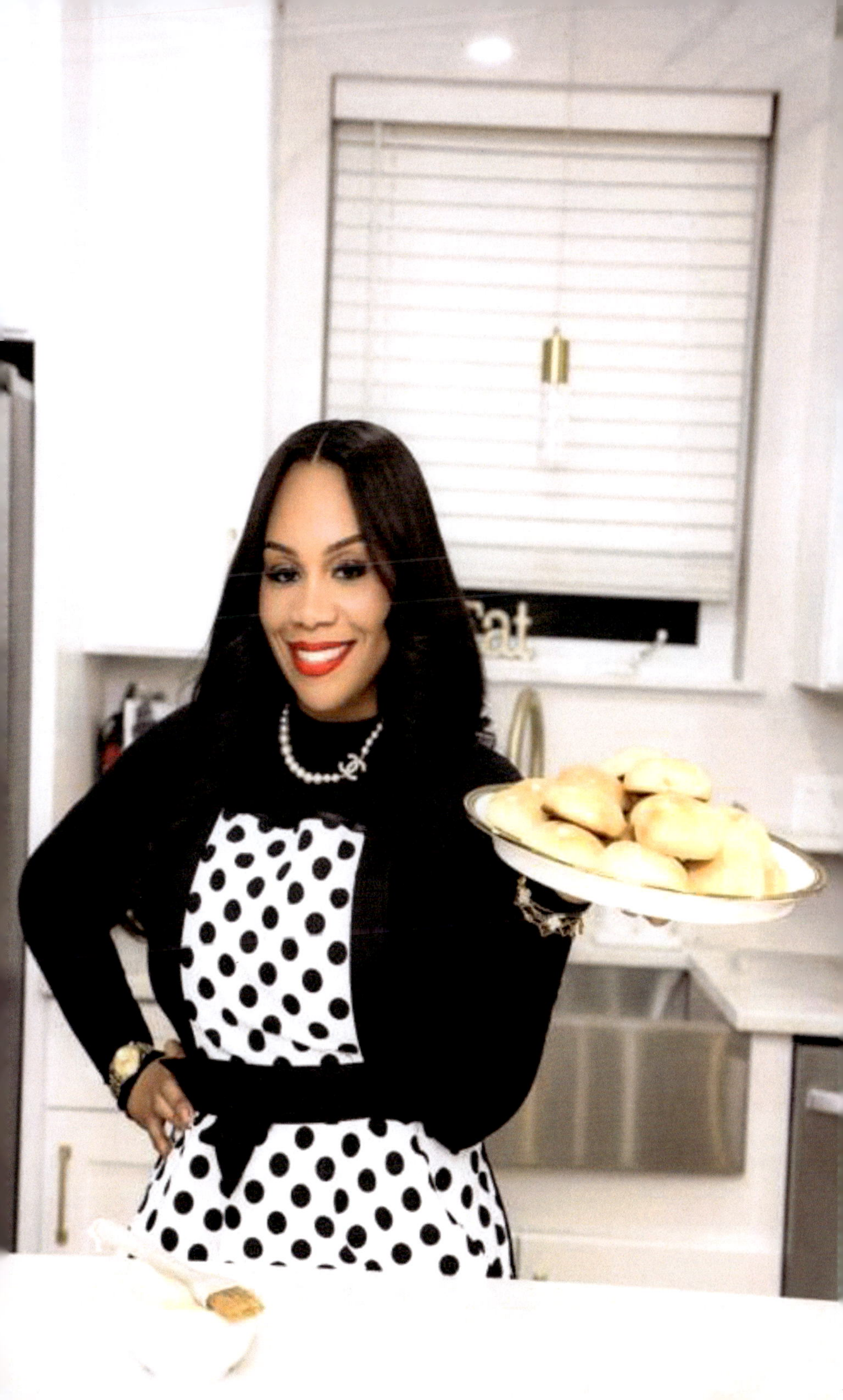

Mac & Cheese

Ingredients

- 4 cups elbow macaroni
- 3 tablespoons salt (for pasta water & seasoning)
- 2 tablespoons flour
- 2 tablespoons ground black pepper
- 2 tablespoons paprika
- ½ stick butter
- 2 tablespoons vegetable oil
- 1 cup Colby Jack cheese
- 1 cup mild cheddar cheese
- 1 cup mozzarella cheese
- 1 cup sharp cheddar cheese
- 3 tablespoons Soulè Secret Seasoning
- 1 cup heavy cream
- 1 cup half-and-half
- 1 cup whole milk

Instructions

1. Cook the Pasta

Bring a pot of water to a boil. Add a pinch of salt and the vegetable oil. Pour in the elbow macaroni and cook until al dente.

Drain the pasta and place it into a baking dish. Set aside.

2. Make the Cheese Sauce

In a saucepan over medium heat, melt the butter. Once melted, whisk in the flour to create a roux.

Slowly pour in the heavy cream, whisking continuously so it stays smooth.

3. Add the Cheese

Add the Colby Jack, mild cheddar, mozzarella, and sharp cheddar cheeses to the saucepan. Whisk until everything melts down and becomes creamy and smooth.

Pour in the half-and-half to thin the sauce just a little.

4. Season It Up

Season the drained macaroni with salt, pepper, Soulè Secret Seasoning, and paprika.

Pour the cheese sauce over the macaroni and stir until everything is fully coated.

Add the whole milk and stir again to loosen the mixture

and keep it creamy.

5. Top & Bake

Sprinkle a little extra cheese over the top for that golden crust.

Bake uncovered at **400°F** for **35 minutes**, or until the top reaches your desired color.

6. Serve

Let it rest for a few minutes, then dig in. Creamy, cheesy, baked to perfection, just how mac & cheese is supposed to be.

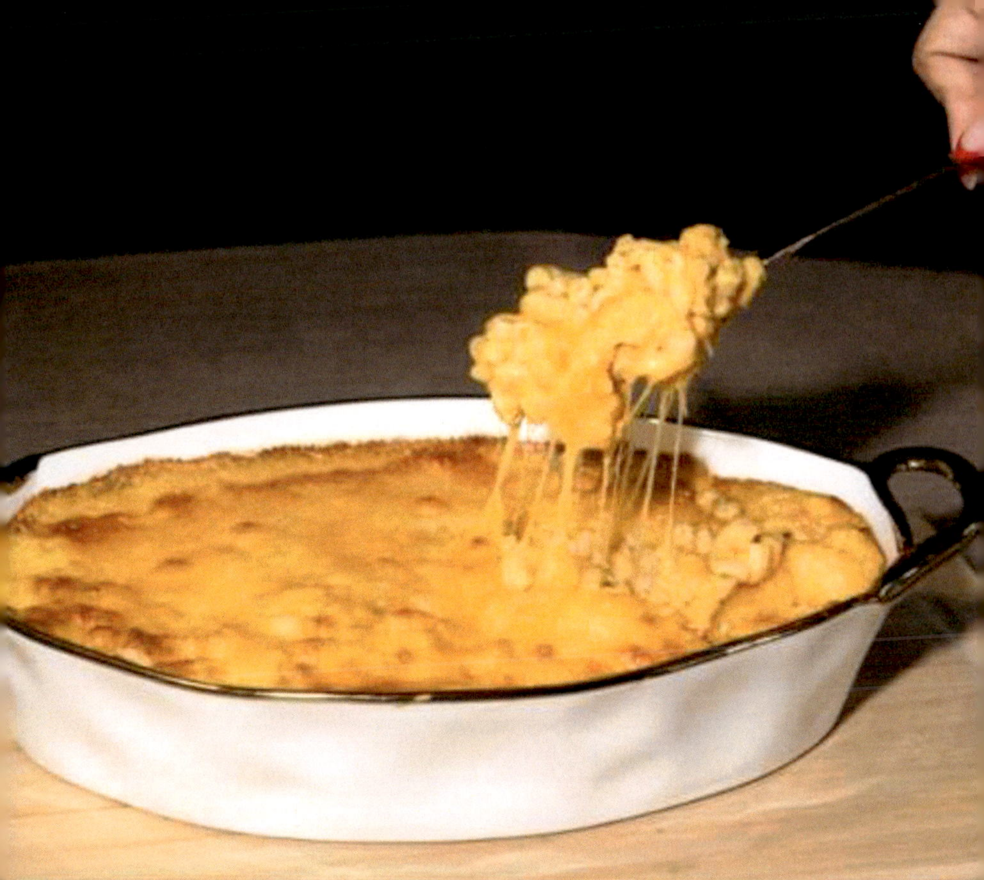

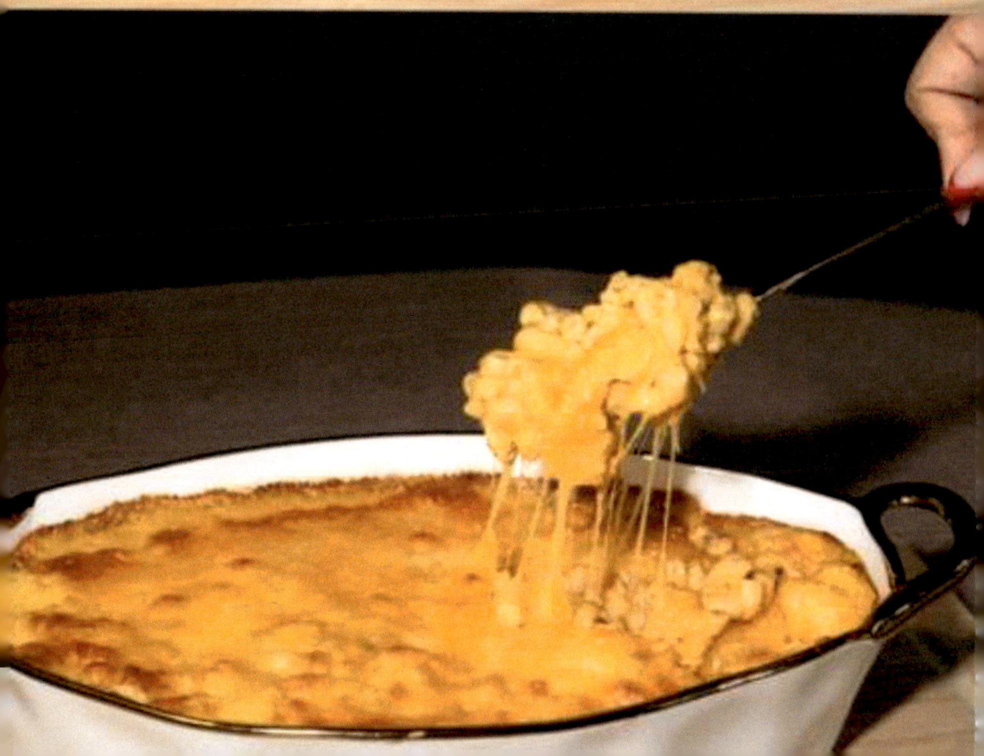

Flat-Footed and Grounded – Red Beans and Rice

Every single day, I was focused on opening that restaurant. I told my friends and family I was opening one, and everybody laughed.

"Girl, you don't know nothing about no restaurant," they'd say.

But I was determined.

People were so used to me starting things and never finishing them. I wore so many hats in my life, y'all have no idea. One minute, I wanted to make belts. I loved a good belt because my grandmother always told me that, since I was heavy in the midsection, I should wear long clothes growing up. I didn't understand it then, but as an adult, I realized she was teaching me how to camouflage my stomach. I was a big girl, almost 300 pounds.

I was a hairstylist. At one point, I even went door-to-door selling knives. I did it all. I've been a hustler my whole life. I sold everything, dreams, wedding rings, you name it. And I always worked a job, too. I've been working since I was 15 years old because I knew I wanted a great life for myself.

The more I practiced my recipes, the better I got. Sunday dinners with my sisters and friends at my childhood home were my practice sessions. I got so good at cooking that it became therapeutic; it was like I was cooking my pain through the food. I wanted to see if people beyond my friends and family would love my food, so I started selling plates on Instagram. I'd whip up a menu on my phone, have my neighbors working the grill, along with my cousin. My nieces handled the phone orders while I cooked up a storm. It was like running a mini-restaurant right out of my mother's kitchen. I got so good at it that I was selling 40-50 plates a day; everyone was loving it!

I had about $50,000 saved, and I just knew that was going to open the doors to my restaurant. I did my research, and they said the average restaurant costs about $150,000 to start.

Chileeee… I knew somebody who knew somebody, so I didn't think it would cost me that much.

I found a small space in Ukrainian Village in Chicago. At first, I didn't even like it, but the more I visited, the more I fell in love. I struggled with the name, but I finally came up with *Soulè*, a fancy way of saying soul. It was going to be a soul food and Creole restaurant, served on fancy dishes. All the soul food spots I knew reminded me of the civil rights movement, and I kept asking myself, why can't soul food be served on porcelain and still be elegant? That was my goal: to switch things up.

When I tell you this journey was one for the books…

That $50,000 was gone before I knew it. I started doing

hair again just to stay afloat. You have to remember, I had just had a conversation with God about saving me from jail, and I was not going back on my word. The Feds still hadn't come knocking, and to this day, I thank God for His grace and mercy because they never did.

This season tested me like never before. I truly felt like God was seeing if He could trust me with the blessing He was about to give me. Everything from my previous life was gone. I was selling my handbags on eBay for pennies on the dollar, my Rolex for crumbs. My family was sad and confused.

"What are you doing? You're going to have nothing."

And they were right, but I was willing to give it all up without hesitation.

I had two kids and a husband, and Sur was helping, too, but I've always been used to being in charge. I was figuring a lot of this out on my own.

People were so used to me having money that they couldn't believe I was broke. I was driving around blocks I used to hang out at, seeing familiar faces, asking dudes, "Let me hold $20." They thought I was joking. I still came outside dressed to impress, broke as a joke. Nobody knew what was behind the makeup.

I sacrificed everything for that restaurant.

I prayed and asked God not just to do this *for* me, but to do this *with* me. I told Him to have His way in my business.

Chileeee… when I tell you God broke me all the way down, He broke me. It felt like a test every single day. It would've been so easy to turn back to the streets, but I stayed on the right track. Once I sold everything, I came up with a little more money, but then, I had to do a full build-out. I don't know if God made it hard on purpose, but I was almost at the finish line and hit another brick wall.

That's when I said, "God, I know you don't want this, but I got one more scam in me."

This time, I wasn't scamming the banks; I was scamming my people. I know how that sounds, but my back was against the wall. It wasn't a full scam, because I did have some of what I promised, just not all.

It was a raffle ticket scam.

I needed my plumbing fixed, and I had no money. Hair was slow, and I didn't know what else to do. I told myself it wasn't as bad because I wasn't throwing rocks at the penitentiary anymore; now, my integrity was on the line.

Sur had two TVs he bought off the street, and I used those as prizes. I promised two TVs and a trip to L.A. My homeboy owned a spa out there, and I asked him if I could name him the winner so people would believe the trip was real. He agreed.

My friends and I hit the streets selling tickets for $10 a pop. I sold $3,000 worth. I took $2,500 and fixed the plumbing. I had $500 left to my name, and I entered a fest to get my name out there.

Here's the crazy part: I didn't even have food to sell at the fest.

I prayed, *Lord, what am I going to do? Why didn't I think about the food?* I knew I had just done some bullshit with the tickets, but in my mind, I was still going to give people something.

Nobody knew I was broke, nobody but my sisters. My ego was too big. I couldn't let the streets know. I called a homeboy who taught me the game, thinking he'd offer me cash. Instead, he offered me 13 stolen credit cards.

I was furious.

"Didn't I just tell you I talked to God? Didn't I just tell you I wasn't living that life anymore?" I hung up the phone, shaking with anger and stress.

That's when I broke down.

I lay on the bathroom floor sobbing, needing my mother. I called my sister, screaming, "She's dead, she's dead."

She said, "Who?"

I said, "Mom."

She replied, "Bridgette… where have you been?"

I had been running from reality. My mother had been dead for eight years, and I never needed her more than I did while trying to open that restaurant. I had no choice but to put my big-girl panties on and keep moving.

I failed my final construction inspection. The same day, I had a meeting with a woman I'd met a year earlier, another restaurant owner. She had always encouraged me and was never a gatekeeper. Everything told me not to go to that meeting, but something pushed me to show up.

She was explaining how to pass my health inspection, the last step before opening, but my mind was everywhere. I didn't tell her what I was going through. All I could think was, I have two days before this fest and nothing to sell.

She got up from the table, left the room, then came back and handed me a check for $500.

She said, "God told me to give this to you."

I will never forget that moment.

I used that $500 to buy food, went to the fest, and made another $2,700. I took that money, got more work done, and before I knew it… my doors were finally on their way to opening.

Moments like that let me know, without a doubt, God is real.

God,

Thank You for always having my back.

Thank You for letting me know that You are real.

Thank You for being an on-time God.

I will continue to be obedient.

Thank You for keeping Your promise to me.

That was my prayer.

Just like red beans and rice, simple, comforting, and rooted in home, I had to strip everything back down to the basics, grounded in faith. I had to get flat-footed and grounded in the process. The raffle, the struggles, even the blessing of that $500. Each step was like building that dish: simple ingredients, but it feeds something bigger. I learned that being firmly planted in faith and perseverance is what finally let everything come together, like my restaurant, born from the most grounded version of me.

Let's get into the Red Beans and Rice!!!

Red Beans & Rice

Ingredients

For the Rice

- 2 cups white rice (or rice in a bag, no judgment)

For the Red Beans

- 6 cups red beans
- 4 cups chicken broth
- 4 smoked turkey tails
- 1 cup diced celery
- 1 cup diced onion
- 1 cup red & green bell peppers, mixed
- 2 bay leaves

Seasonings

- 2 tablespoons cumin
- 1 tablespoon Creole seasoning
- 1 tablespoon Cajun seasoning
- 2 tablespoons Soulè Secret Seasoning
- 1 teaspoon sugar

• 1 teaspoon ground black pepper

Instructions

1. Make the Rice First

Let's start with the rice. Baby… I don't know how to boil rice to save my life, so I use **rice in a bag**.

I know I probably shouldn't have said that, but I like to keep it real.

If you use a rice cooker or have your own way of making rice, go right ahead and do you.

2. Boil the Smoked Turkey

In a large stock pot, bring the smoked turkey tails to a boil.

Cook until they're nice and tender, and that smoky flavor is all up in the broth.

3. Build the Beans

Once the turkey tails are soft, add in:

• Red beans

• Chicken broth

• Bay leaves

• Bell peppers, onion, and celery

4. Season It Up

Add all your seasonings:

- Sugar
- Black pepper
- Soulè Secret Seasoning
- Cumin
- Cajun seasoning
- Creole seasoning

Stir everything together well.

5. Cook Low & Slow

Let the beans cook for about **1½ hours**, stirring occasionally.

Taste as you go, and if you feel like it needs more seasoning, **add it**.

You already know… we season as we go.

6. Serve

Spoon those rich, flavorful red beans over a bed of rice and enjoy.

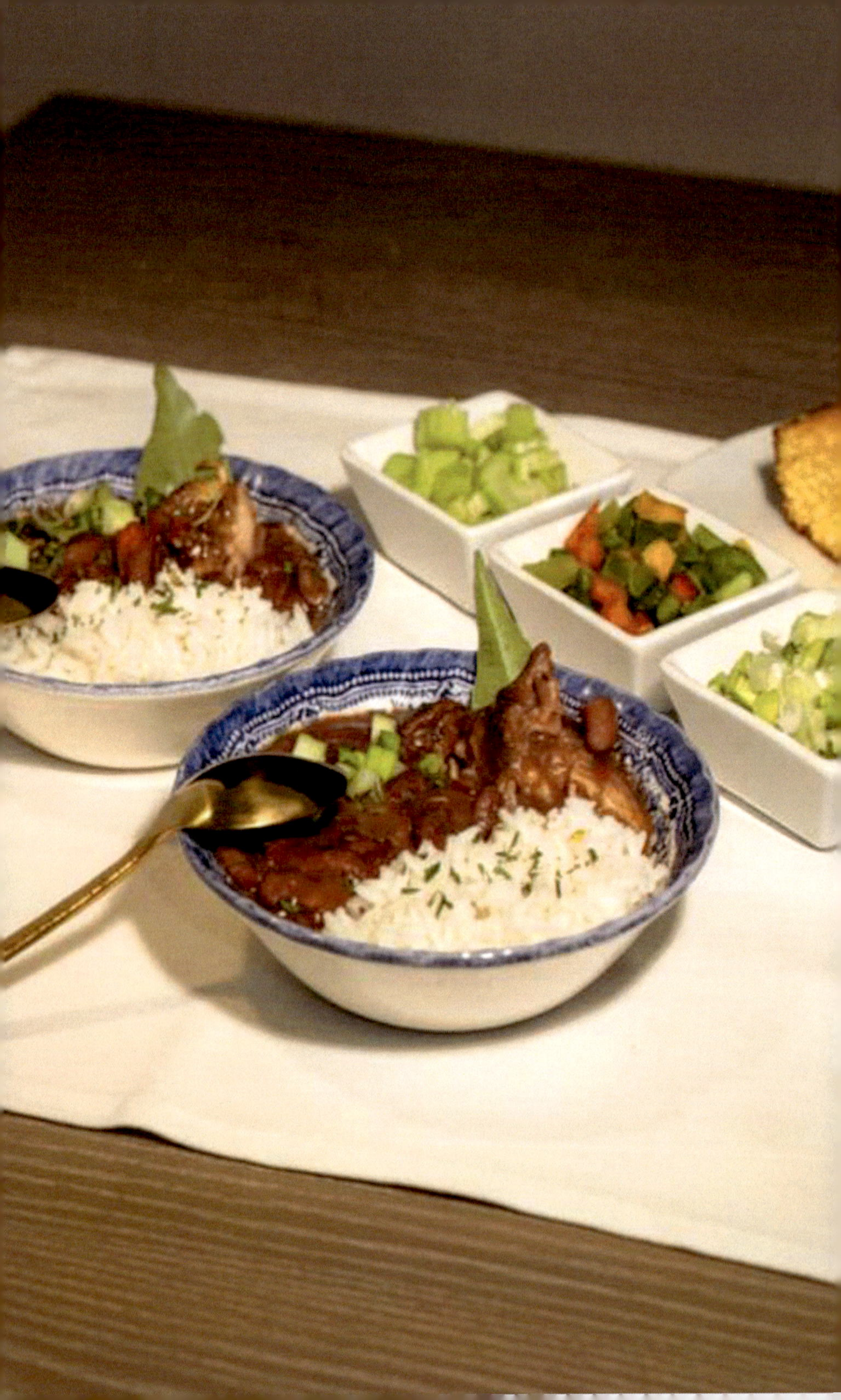

The String Bean Queen – String Beans with Smoked Turkey & White Potatoes

As the restaurant was about to open, I found myself reflecting.

Cooking has always been in my blood. My grandmother, a phenomenal cook, was the head chef at a Chicago public school. When I say she could cook everything, I mean everything. She left big shoes to fill.

My mother could cook, too. I come from a family that loved to entertain and care for people. My grandmother came to Chicago during the Great Migration, from Panthers Burn to Greenwood, Mississippi. She'd open her doors to newcomers from the South, help them get on their feet, and send them on their way. My family-owned taverns, hosted parties, and kept doors open to all. I guess that's where I get it from, feeding people, giving what I have, even my last.

When I imagine my restaurant, I envision family. I want to bring family back into the community because it's missing. Opening this restaurant will change my life, and I hope it changes the lives of those who work with me.

As I cooked more, I got better. I've mentioned tacos, but the first dish I truly learned was green beans, which my mom taught me before she passed. Every weekend, I'd cook those green beans to bring the family together. I didn't know how to fry chicken yet, so I'd buy some and serve it with my mom's famous green beans. Sundays were for practicing with my sisters and their kids, Bobby Womack playing, as I mimicked my mom and grandmother. I wanted that smell to be just like I remembered. My family called me the *String Bean Queen* because, well, that's all I knew how to cook.

Those kitchen moments reminded me of family, something I miss. I didn't realize how precious that time was. I didn't take time to make time, and I ran out of time. I thought they would be here forever.

That string bean recipe was the start of a great future for me. My mother and I cooked a lot of different dishes together, but for some reason, that was the only recipe I could ever remember, and it meant everything to me. That recipe brought my family back together. It turned friends into family. It will forever live in my heart because it was a piece of my mother. I'd cook those green beans to bring the family back together after she died.

When I finally mastered that dish, I was so proud. I wanted everybody to eat it. I used to just sit back and watch people while they ate, watching their faces light up, watching them smile. I cooked with love, and seeing people enjoy my food gave me real satisfaction. I wasn't just cooking anymore; I was cooking with a purpose.

So when my family started calling me the *String Bean Queen*, I felt like I earned that name. Those string beans had a piece of my soul in them.

That string bean recipe carried way more than flavor for me. It carried my mama. It carried my family, my memories, and a time when we were all still together. Every time I cooked it, it felt like I was holding on to something I didn't want to lose. It brought people to the table, started conversations, and filled spaces that needed love.

That dish reminded me why I cook, and why food means so much to me. This wasn't just something I learned how to make. It was something I felt.

Thank You, God, for the vision You've blessed me with.

Thank You for my family and the seeds of love and strength they planted in me.

Thank You for the love they poured into my life and the love they served to others, one plate at a time.

So let me show you how I make the recipe that will always have a piece of my heart in it, the one that made me the *String Bean Queen.*

Green Beans with Smoked Turkey & Potatoes

Ingredients

- 6 smoked turkey necks
- 5 bags fresh green beans (or frozen cut green beans, if needed)
- 4 white potatoes, peeled and cut
- ½ white onion, diced
- 1 stick butter
- 2 tablespoons salt
- 2 tablespoons black pepper
- 3 tablespoons chicken soup base

Instructions

Let's get into it, because this right here is **my favorite recipe**.

This was the **first dish I ever learned how to cook**, so it'll always hit different.

1. Boil the Smoked Turkey

In a large stock pot, bring the smoked turkey necks to a boil.

Let them cook until the meat starts releasing that good,

smoky flavor into the broth.

2. Prep the Green Beans

While the turkey is boiling, rinse your green beans and **pick them**.

Yes, it's time-consuming. I like to cut the ends off each one and slice them down the middle.

If you don't have the time, it's perfectly fine to use frozen cut green beans.

3. Build the Pot

Add the green beans to the pot with the turkey necks.

Then add the potatoes, diced onion, salt, pepper, and chicken soup base.

Drop the stick of butter right on top.

4. Simmer Low & Slow

Stir everything together, cover the pot, and let it simmer for about **45 minutes**, stirring occasionally.

5. Serve

Once the green beans are tender, the potatoes are soft, and the broth is rich, you're done.

And when I tell you **this is a game-changer for green beans**, believe me.

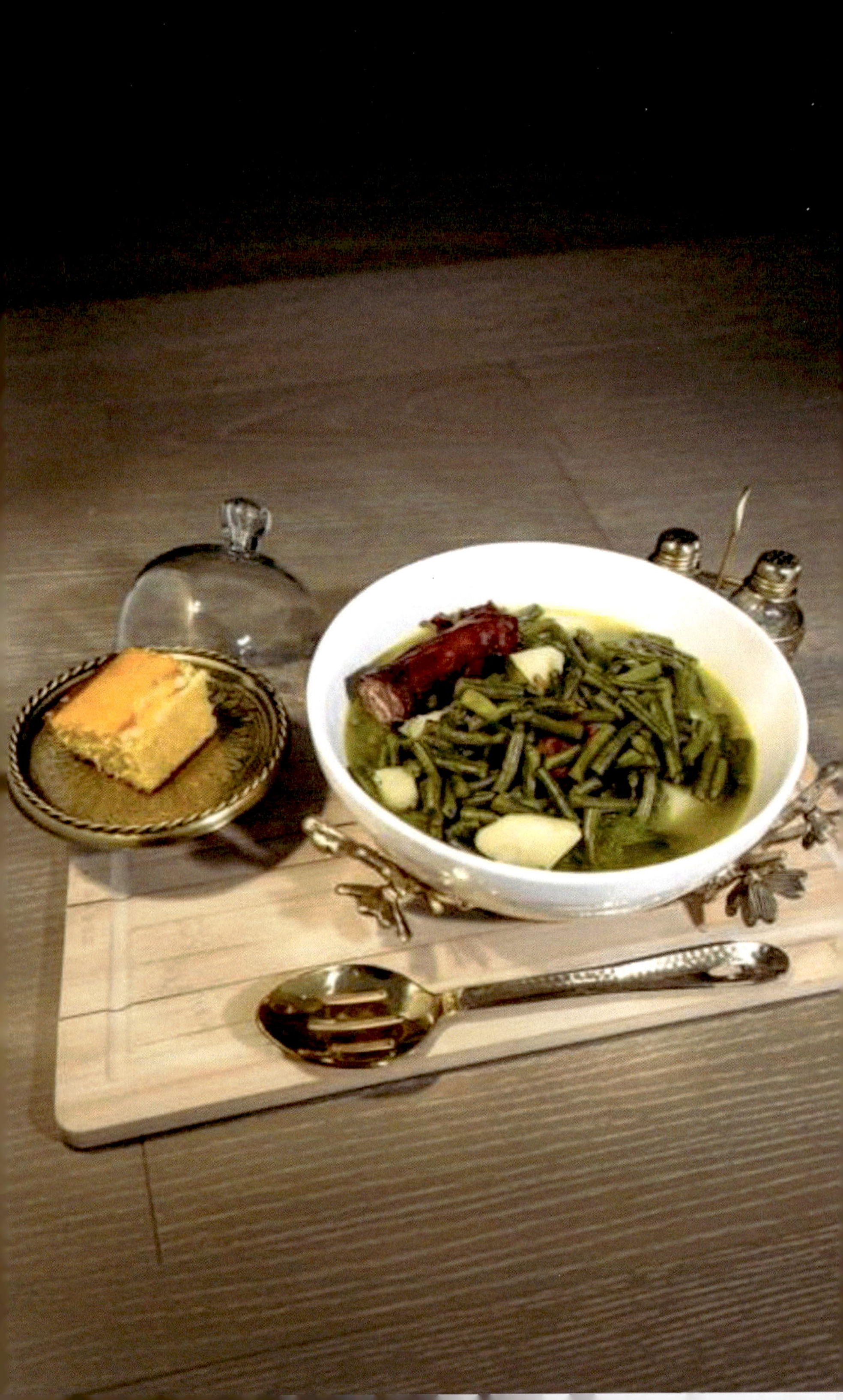

Life Is Peachy – Peach Cobbler

I couldn't believe how my life had transformed over that year and a half. When I signed the lease in June 2016, I had no idea that from then until October 2017, I'd feel like I was living through my own Job moment. God took me through the wringer, but I never lost my faith. I believed He was testing me, seeing if I could be trusted with the blessing He had in store.

During that time, I stayed still, obedient, and held onto my promise. There were moments of fear being on the straight and narrow when I was used to having money, but I kept thinking of the promise I made to God. His word says *He will never leave you nor forsake you*, and during that year and a half of building that restaurant, He didn't leave me once.

Throughout those years, I had made my share of bad decisions. It often felt like life had defeated me, like I was getting my ass kicked by men, women, and my own choices. But I'm so grateful that I changed my way of thinking. Changing my mind changed my life.

I wanted to make my family proud, to earn everything by doing right. I wanted to be the granddaughter who honored her grandmother's strength, the daughter who made her father proud, even if I didn't finish college, and the daughter my mother could rely on to be strong. I wanted to be an honest, hardworking mother and a role model for my kids, showing them that their start didn't have to be their finish. I wanted to inspire young people from my community to rise above their circumstances.

When all my inspections were finally passed, and it was time for the grand opening, I could hardly believe it. *Soulè* was finally here. God had stripped away everything from my past life, the unearned money, the material things, and left me with just enough to serve food to my community at the opening. I couldn't even afford new outfits for the kids and me. But none of that mattered.

Friends and family never really knew what I was going through. My pride was loud, my ego even louder, and I refused to let anyone see me struggle. But life has a funny way of humbling you, especially when you think you've got everything under control.

I remember the day of the grand opening. I had so many doubts about myself. It felt like the devil was sitting right there, planting fear in my heart, trying to pull me back into my old life.

Am I good enough? Am I smart enough? I'm not formally trained. Will I even make it in this industry? This is a tough business. And I kept asking myself: *how did I even have the balls to open a restaurant with no real knowledge, nothing but a dream?*

Then it hit me. I had the balls to do all the wrong things

in life. I took risks when it didn't make sense. So if I could be that bold doing wrong, I had to believe that when I finally chose to do something right… something positive had to come from it.

My friends and family showed up in droves. They helped cook, serve, and made the day unforgettable. That morning, I prayed and asked God to enter my business and my life fully, to have His way. I opened *Soulè* with a prayer and the only batch of food I could afford, but I was proud and at peace.

For the first time, I stuck with something and saw it through. For once, I wasn't looking over my shoulder. Life was peachy because I had peace, and I had God on my side. I wasn't chasing validation from anyone or anything.

I was no longer running into the arms of men, chasing that high of the love my father once gave me. I was no longer throwing rocks at the penitentiary. I was no longer a product of my environment. I wasn't living recklessly anymore, and I wasn't running from my reality. I was embracing it, and it felt just right.

Life was finally peachy, and I had found my peace. Just like a perfectly baked peach cobbler, life had a mix of sweet and challenging layers, each one adding depth and richness to the flavor. Every challenge, every setback, and every triumph added a layer of depth and flavor to my journey. It all came together to create something beautiful, something worth savoring.

And just like this journey, my peach cobbler recipe carries the essence of resilience, comfort, and the sweetness of new beginnings. Let each bite remind you that no matter how tough the journey, the end result can be as sweet and fulfilling as a warm, golden dessert.

Peach Cobbler

Ingredients

• 4 pie crusts (use as needed, depending on dish size)

• 4 cans sliced peaches in heavy syrup

• 1 stick butter, sliced

• 2 tablespoons nutmeg

• 2 tablespoons cinnamon

• ½ cup imitation vanilla

• 1 cup granulated sugar

• 2 tablespoons light brown sugar

Instructions

Let's get into this peach cobbler.

1. Make the Filling

In a saucepan, pour in the peaches (with the syrup).

Add:

• Nutmeg

• Cinnamon

• Imitation vanilla

- Granulated sugar
- Butter

Stir everything together until the butter is melted and the peaches are coated in that good syrupy flavor.

Taste it. Make sure it's sweet enough *before* you pour it.

2. Prep the Baking Dish

In a baking dish, line the bottom with pie crust.

Depending on the size of your dish, you may need:

- one crust on the bottom and one on top
- or two on the bottom and two on top

Do what works best for your pan.

3. Assemble the Cobbler

Pour the peach filling over the bottom crust.

Sprinkle the light brown sugar evenly over the peaches.

Place the remaining pie crust on top.

4. Bake

Bake at **375°F** until golden brown, about **30–45 minutes**, depending on your oven.

5. Serve

Let it cool just a little… then dig in.

And there you have it, **Life Is Peachy Peach Cobbler.**

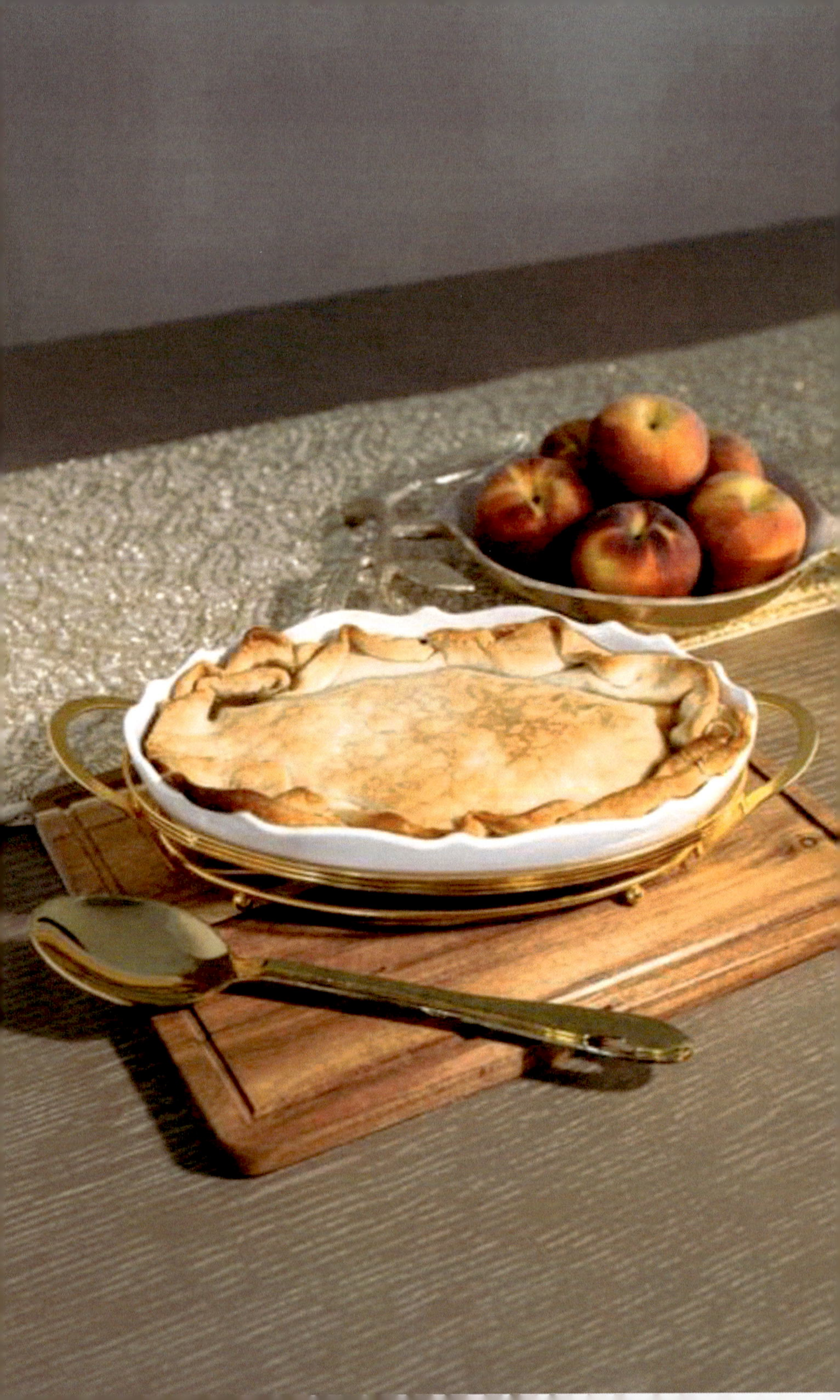

Closing Prayer

Thank You, Lord, for never giving up on me.

Thank You for Your grace and Your mercy.

Thank You for being a fence around me every day,

especially on the days when I was doing wrong.

Thank You for changing my life.

Thank You for my ups and my downs,

for the lessons and for all my blessings.

Thank You for making a way out of no way.

Thank You for my family, my friends, and my community,

for everyone who helped shape me into the strong, resilient woman I am today.

Thank You for my mother, my grandmother, and my father.

And God, if You never do another thing for me,

You have already done enough.

www.ingramcontent.com/pod-product-compliance
Ingram Content Group UK Ltd.
Pitfield, Milton Keynes, MK11 3LW, UK
UKRC030246051026
15591UKWH00007BA/344

* 9 7 8 1 9 6 8 7 3 2 4 6 2 *

9 781968 732462